ASK YOUR DOCTOR
ABOUT CELEBREX™

- If you're unable to get pain relief from other medications
- If aspirin or other pain medicines irritate your stomach
- If the pain and swelling of arthritis are limiting your activities
- If real pain relief is the miracle you've been looking for

CELEBREX™
MAY BE YOUR ANSWER
THIS BOOK WILL MAKE YOU
AN INFORMED CONSUMER

D1636777

ATTENTION: ORGANIZATIONS AND CORPORATIONS
Most Avon Books paperbacks are available at special quantity
discounts for bulk purchases for sales promotions, premiums, or
fund-raising. For information, please call or write:

**Special Markets Department, HarperCollins Publishers Inc.
10 East 53rd Street, New York, New York 10022-5299.
Telephone: (212) 207-7528.   Fax: (212) 207-7222.**

CELEBREX™

Cox-2 Inhibitors—
The Amazing
New Pain Fighters

Shelagh Ryan Masline
Foreword by Jay Goldstein, M.D.

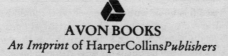

AVON BOOKS
An Imprint of HarperCollins*Publishers*

CELEBREX is not a substitute for sound medical advice. The ideas, procedures, and suggestions in this book are intended to supplement, not replace, the medical advice of a trained medical professional. All matters regarding your health require medical supervision. Consult your physician before adopting the suggestions in this book, as well as about any condition that may require diagnosis or medical attention. The author and publisher disclaim any liability arising directly or indirectly from the use of this book.

Celebrex™ is a registered trademark of G.D. Searle & Company, a division of Monsanto Company.

AVON BOOKS
An Imprint of HarperCollins*Publishers*
10 East 53rd Street
New York, New York 10022-5299

Copyright © 1999 by Shelagh Ryan Masline
Library of Congress Catalog Card Number: 99-94455
ISBN: 0-380-80897-8
www.avonbooks.com

All rights reserved. No part of this book may be used or reproduced in any manner whatsoever without written permission, except in the case of brief quotations embodied in critical articles and reviews. For information address Avon Books, an imprint of HarperCollins Publishers.

First WholeCare printing: November 1999

Avon Trademark Reg. U.S. Pat. Off. and in Other Countries, Marca Registrada, Hecho en U.S.A.
HarperCollins® is a trademark of HarperCollins Publishers Inc.

Printed in the U.S.A.

20   19   18   17   16   15   14   13   12   11   10   9

If you purchased this book without a cover, you should be aware that this book is stolen property. It was reported as "unsold and destroyed" to the publisher, and neither the author nor the publisher has received any payment for this "stripped book."

*To my mother Eileen,
in hopes that she will soon
take advantage of this wonderful new medication*

Acknowledgments

The author would like to take this opportunity to acknowledge the many others who contributed to this book. Many thanks to Jay L. Goldstein, M.D., associate professor of medicine at the University of Illinois at Chicago and medical director of clinical resource management at the University of Illinois Hospital and Clinics, for reviewing this manuscript and providing the Foreword. I'm also very grateful to Peter C. Isakson, M.D., who leads COX-2 Technology Research and Development at Searle, for taking the time to discuss COX-2 inhibitors with me and to review portions of the manuscript. Thanks to my agent, Judith Riven, and to Dr. Selwyn Cohen for providing me with my first glimpses of Celebrex. Many folks who participated in the Celebrex clinical trials were kind enough to share their experiences with me, including Frank Edwards, Shirley Johnson, Anne Pollack, Laurie Schuster, and Laurie Stollery. I'm grateful to Beth Keshishian at the Chandler Chicco Agency for arranging these interviews and providing support in other logistical matters. And last but not least, thanks to my editor at Avon Books, Ann McKay Thoroman, and her invaluable assistant, Sarah Durand.

Contents

◆◆◆◆

Foreword by Jay Goldstein, M.D.   xi

PART I: ARTHRITIS: DEFINITIONS AND OVERVIEW

Chapter One: What Is Arthritis?   3

Chapter Two: What Kind of Arthritis Do
You Have?   23

Chapter Three: Standard Drug Therapy
for Arthritis   63

PART II: THE COX-2 INHIBITOR SOLUTION

Chapter Four: The History of
COX-2 Inhibitors   97

Chapter Five: COX-2 Inhibitors:
The Stomach-Friendly Alternative   108

Chapter Six: Managing the Pain   136

PART III: NATURAL TREATMENTS FOR ARTHRITIS

Chapter Seven: Diet and Arthritis   169

Chapter Eight: The Anti-Arthritis
    Exercise Program   199

Chapter Nine: Managing Your
    Day-to-Day Activities   227

Chapter Ten: Alternative Treatments
    for Arthritis   244

Glossary   269

Appendix A: Further Resources   279

Appendix B: Further Information   281

Bibliography   283

Index   285

Foreword

Approximately 40 million Americans suffer from osteoarthritis and rheumatoid arthritis and many others have various inflammatory disorders that require the use of medication for the relief of pain and inflammation. It is estimated that in excess of $5 billion is spent annually in the United States for the treatment of patients with arthritis. These costs arise from the direct monies spent to provide medical care, as well as a much larger amount that is associated with the inability to work, and lost wages as a result of arthritis-associated disabilities. While medical research has made great advances in treating the underlying causes of various arthritic conditions, the American public is still burdened with the cost of care and disability related to arthritis. In other words, we still have tremendous opportunities to apply these research efforts into the daily practice of medicine.

Nonsteroidal anti-inflammatory drugs (NSAIDs) have long been a mainstay for the treatment of pain and inflammatory conditions. It is estimated that 17% of the American population uses these types of medications for the treatment of inflammatory disorders and painful syndromes. While these medications are effective and widely used, they are not without risk. By the same mechanism that they reduce inflammation, these medications are associated with gastrointestinal side effects including pain, ulcers, and ulcer complications, most notably ulcer bleeding. Unfortunately, many Americans are unaware of these complications and use these medications freely with little knowledge about their adverse complications.

In a recent survey, approximately 75% of patients using nonsteroidal anti-inflammatory drugs were either unaware or unconcerned about the complications associated with these treatments. This is again quite unfortunate since the average annual risk for developing complications related to the use of these medications is estimated to be between 2% and 4% for continuous nonsteroidal users. Furthermore, patients with a past history of ulcers, those using higher doses of these medications, and notably the elderly are more prone to developing complications on NSAIDs with annual rates of complications annually occurring in up to 10% of these high-risk patients. In 1998 it was estimated that there were over 100,000 hospitalizations related to complications of the use of nonsteroidal anti-inflammatory drugs. What is even more striking is the fact that over 10% of patients who sustain a complication related to the use of these medications will die as a result. While educational programs are directed to better educate the American population, these endeavors often fall short of reducing these serious and life-threatening complications associated with the use of NSAIDs.

Approximately eight years ago a major change in

our understanding of the use of anti-inflammatory agents was identified in the laboratory. We now recognize, based on these studies, that the adverse effects of traditional nonsteroidal anti-inflammatory drugs can be averted. All nonsteroidal anti-inflammatory drugs inhibit an enzyme called cyclooxygenase. This enzyme is found in the stomach as well as at the site of inflammation. At the site of inflammation, inhibition of cyclooxygenase results in pain relief and an anti-inflammatory effect. This enzyme, however, is also found in the stomach and the intestine and is responsible for maintaining a protective barrier against injury to the gastrointestinal lining. By using medications such as NSAIDs that block this enzyme, patients are predisposed to ulcers and the complications of ulcer disease.

The discovery in the laboratory that has revolutionized our approach to anti-inflammatory therapies was quite simple yet elegant. We now recognize that cyclooxygenase is actually present in two forms. The form in the stomach is called cyclooxygenase-1 (COX 1) and the form at the sites of inflammation is called COX 2. Biochemical analysis has allowed scientists to develop new medications that selectively block COX 2, but spare the activity and function of COX 1. In doing so, these medications known as COX-2 inhibitors, are anti-inflammatory and cause pain relief without predisposing to the development of ulcers in the GI lining. This finding has provided a very important advancement in safety for the treatment of patients with arthritis. Clinicians worldwide are optimistic that this new class of agents, called COX-2 inhibitors, will provide arthritis sufferers the anti-inflammatory and analgesic effect that we clinically desire, but without gastrointestinal toxicity and ulcer complications.

This book was written to better educate patients with arthritis and to integrate the knowledge we know about anti-inflammatory drugs. Armed with better knowledge, arthritis sufferers can better co-participate with their physicians and healthcare providers in the management of their painful and inflammatory disorders. It is exciting to see the rapid evolution of arthritis care be translated from the laboratory to the "bedside" and into daily medical practice. It is anticipated that the advances made by the use of specific COX-2 inhibitors will benefit millions of patients annually.

Jay Goldstein, M.D.
Associate Professor of Medicine
Section of Digestive and Liver Diseases
The University of Illinois at Chicago

PART I

ARTHRITIS:
DEFINITIONS AND OVERVIEW

ONE

✦✦✦✦

What Is Arthritis?

Not too long ago I was walking with a cane. But now that I'm taking Celebrex, I feel much better. This past New Year's Eve, I even went out and danced. My cane has been retired to the corner now, and I'm going to bring it to my church and donate it to somebody who really needs it.

Laurie Schuster, 37-year-old osteoarthritis patient
and participant in Celebrex clinical trials

Chances are that you or someone close to you suffers from arthritis, a sometimes crippling joint disease that affects nearly one in six Americans. For the more than 40 million people in this country who struggle with one form of arthritis or another, a wide variety of medications and techniques are available to manage pain, stiffness, and swelling. But it is an unfortunate reality that many medications potentially have unpleasant and sometimes even dangerous side effects. Because of this, scientists are constantly exploring new avenues in the treatment of this troubling family of disorders.

In this book you will learn about an exciting new group of anti-arthritis medications called COX-2 inhibitors. Celebrex, or celecoxib (its generic name), is the first FDA-approved COX-2 inhibitor. Not everybody who takes Celebrex throws away her cane and goes out dancing like Laurie Schuster, but many have found welcome relief from pain and inflammation coupled with a wonderful new freedom from side effects. In clinical trials involving thousands of arthritis patients, therapeutic doses of Celebrex reduced pain and inflammation as effectively as ibuprofen and similar medications while causing fewer gastrointestinal side effects such as bleeding ulcers.

What is arthritis?

The word *arthritis* comes from the Greek *arth*, which means "joint," and *itis*, which means "inflammation." Arthritis is actually an umbrella term for more than 100 different diseases that affect primarily the joints but sometimes other parts of the body as well. Most frequently, arthritic or rheumatic diseases involve pain, stiffness, and in many cases inflammation of the joints. Joints are the junctions at which bones come together, such as at the knees and hips.

How common is arthritis?

Arthritis affects nearly one in six Americans, or more than 40 million people. This represents 15 percent of the population of the United States. With the aging of the baby boomer generation, the number of people who have arthritis is expected to reach 60 million by the year 2020. Worldwide, some 350 million people suffer from arthritis.

What types of arthritis are new COX-2 inhibitors designed to treat?

At present COX-2 inhibitors have been approved by the Food and Drug Administration (FDA) for the treatment of osteoarthritis and adult rheumatoid arthritis. It is possible that in time they will be prescribed to treat other types of arthritis. In addition, the FDA approved Vioxx for the treatment of acute general and menstrual pain. (Vioxx has *not* yet been approved for the treatment of rheumatoid arthritis.)

What are the most common types of arthritis?

Osteoarthritis and rheumatoid arthritis are most common. In osteoarthritis (OA), cartilage deteriorates over time in the hips, knees, feet, and spine. In rheumatoid arthritis (RA), the membranes lining the joints become inflamed, limiting the joint's range of motion. RA is an autoimmune disease, caused when the body mistakenly attacks its own tissues. OA may affect just one joint, while RA usually affects many joints.

How many people suffer from these types of arthritis?

In this country, about 21 million people have osteoarthritis, and more than 2 million suffer from rheumatoid arthritis. Worldwide, nearly 190 million individuals have osteoarthritis, and more than 16.5 million have rheumatoid arthritis. Related problems such as gout, lupus, fibromyalgia, and osteoporosis frequently occur as well. (Read more about the many different types of arthritis and related conditions in Chapter Two.)

What makes COX-2 inhibitors different from other drugs prescribed to treat arthritis?

COX-2 inhibitors are as effective in relieving joint pain and inflammation as ibuprofen and other non-steroidal anti-inflammatory drugs, or NSAIDs, but in therapeutic doses they reduce the incidence of uncomfortable and sometimes life-threatening side effects such as ulcers and stomach bleeding.

What are NSAIDs?

NSAIDs are the most commonly prescribed medications for arthritis. As their name states, they are drugs that are not steroids but do control inflammation. NSAIDs also control pain.

Are there a number of different COX-2 inhibitors?

Yes. Celebrex was only the first FDA-approved COX-2 inhibitor, shortly followed by Vioxx. Others are still under review. COX-2 inhibitors, members of a special subcategory of NSAIDs, are more selective in their actions in our bodies than ordinary NSAIDs, and because of this they cause fewer gastrointestinal side effects.

Do COX-2 inhibitors have any other potential uses?

Yes. Researchers believe COX-2 inhibitors may play a role in the prevention of colon cancer and Alzheimer's disease, and in the reduction of many types of pain. These include dental pain, menstrual cramps, postsurgical discomfort, backaches, and headaches. In Chapter Four we will take a much closer, in-depth look at COX-2 inhibitors, but first let's examine the disease they are especially designed to treat.

Who is likely to develop arthritis?

Arthritis affects people of all ages in all walks of life, and it appears in countries around the world. It strikes men, women, and even children. Different types of arthritis target different groups of individuals. For example:

- In **osteoarthritis**, the most common form of this disease, decades of wear and tear on the joints eventually lead to the breakdown of bones and cartilage, causing pain and stiffness. Mostly men and women over fifty suffer from OA.

- **Rheumatoid arthritis**, a very serious autoimmune disease of unknown origin, can lead to irreversible joint and organ damage. It most commonly occurs in women between the ages of 25 and 50.

- **Gout** is a very painful form of arthritis that usually affects the big toes, ankles, and knees. It most commonly occurs in men, often beginning around middle age.

- **Lupus**, an autoimmune disease that causes inflammation in the joints and other internal organs, is most common in women, particularly during their childbearing years. It frequently occurs in African Americans.

- **Fibromyalgia**, a syndrome of chronic aching pain, stiffness, and tenderness in the muscles, tendons, and ligaments, is much more common in women than men. It usually occurs between the ages of 20 and 50.

- **Osteoporosis**, a disease of increasingly fragile bones, leads to more than a million fractures each year. It is most common in postmenopausal women, especially small-framed Caucasians and Asians.

Do women develop arthritis more frequently than men?

About two thirds—or 23 million—of the Americans who have arthritis are women.

I've heard that arthritis is just an inevitable part of growing older. Is that true?

No. Some older people are lucky enough to escape arthritis altogether, while certain types of arthritis are more prevalent in young people.

How can I tell whether or not I am suffering from arthritis?

The most common warning signs of this disease are:

- Pain
- Stiffness
- Inflammation or swelling
- Trouble moving a joint

Are the warning signs of arthritis always the same?

No, they're not. The different types of arthritis and related conditions manifest themselves in a number of different ways. Sometimes symptoms come on suddenly, but in other cases they develop slowly over time. Pain can be either constant or intermittent. It may occur only in certain parts of your body, or you may find yourself aching all over. Arthritis sufferers may find stiffness and pain to be especially pronounced in the morning, after being physically inactive for a period of time, or after overdoing physical activity. In a few cases, arthritis is most troublesome when you're lying perfectly still.

Is arthritis always accompanied by inflammation?

Not always. Osteoarthritis is due to wear and tear and very often does not involve inflammation. On the other hand, rheumatoid arthritis is an inflammatory disease involving redness, warmth, and swelling of the skin over an affected joint.

In addition to RA, are there other common types of inflammatory arthritis?

Other common inflammatory conditions include lupus and gout.

My knees have been bothering me when I climb the stairs. Should I see my doctor?

Absolutely. Whenever you experience pain, stiffness, inflammation, or trouble moving a joint for more than two weeks, it's important to make an appointment with your doctor. Only your doctor can tell you whether or not you are suffering from arthritis, what type of arthritis you have, and how it should be treated.

Why do people sometimes delay in seeking treatment for arthritis?

There are many reasons for this. Some keep hoping that if they just ignore pain and stiffness, it will go away. Others are worried about medical coverage. But in many cases delaying treatment can lead to more extensive damage and debility. Over time inflammation can have a cumulative and potentially irreversible effect on your joints.

What causes arthritis?

The causes of most types of arthritis remain unknown. Keep in mind too that there are more than 100 types of arthritis and related conditions, and there can be a correspondingly wide variety of contributing factors. But the good news is that even when causes remain elusive, effective treatments are available.

What are some of the factors that contribute to developing arthritis?

Three factors are most important:

1. Genes

2. Lifestyle

3. Environment

Is it possible to prevent arthritis?

Unfortunately, you can't change your genetic makeup. This means that if arthritis runs in your family, you are more likely to develop it. But there are many steps you can take to reduce your risk of developing this disease.

What can I do to help prevent arthritis?

There are no 100% guarantees, but making certain adjustments to your lifestyle—such as eating healthy foods, getting regular exercise, maintaining an appropriate weight, and managing stress—can reduce your risk of developing arthritis and your degree of disability if you already suffer from this disease.

How does controlling my weight help lower my risk of developing arthritis?

Not surprisingly, excess weight places excess pressure on your joints. This makes it particularly important to maintain a sensible weight, especially as you grow older. Middle-aged and older women who lose 11 pounds over a 10-year period reduce their risk of developing knee arthritis by as much as 50%, according to the Arthritis Foundation.

Do infections cause arthritis?

Infections are involved with some types of arthritis. For example, Lyme disease is caused by being bitten by a deer tick infected with the Lyme virus. Although there is no proof of this, many scientists also believe that rheumatoid arthritis can be triggered by an infection. Most susceptible are people whose immune systems have been compromised by diseases such as diabetes or other forms of arthritis, or who are taking medication for problems such as cancer, hepatitis, or HIV.

If an infection can cause arthritis, does this mean that arthritis is contagious?

Absolutely not. Arthritis is not a contagious disease.

My mother always told me that cracking my knuckles would give me arthritis. Is that true?

No. This is one of the many myths surrounding arthritis. Other myths concern cures for the disease.

Is there a cure for arthritis?

No, but there are many ways to manage arthritis.

People tell me that arthritis is a chronic disease. What does this mean?

Chronic means that you have a disease for a long period of time. It is the opposite of *acute*. Although its symptoms may come and go, once you have arthritis you have it for life. Medication and other treatments can alleviate pain and inflammation and slow its destructive course, but they cannot cure arthritis.

How is arthritis treated?

There are many drugs designed to control the symptoms of arthritis. These now include COX-2 inhibitors such as Celebrex and Vioxx, new NSAIDs that in therapeutic doses can relieve joint pain and inflammation while causing fewer gastrointestinal side effects. Beyond medication, many other treatments are available. For example, physical and occupational therapy can relieve pain and swelling, increase or retain your range of motion, and help you learn how to cope with your disease. Relaxation techniques such as meditation and visualization can be practiced to manage the pain and stress associated with arthritis.

Do support groups play any role in treatment?

They can. Many people who have arthritis join support groups for social and emotional support and to share their experiences with others who suffer from similar problems. It's very important not to allow yourself to become isolated and depressed when you have a chronic disease. Support groups, which are available through the Arthritis Foundation, are also a good forum in which to swap self-care tips and to keep abreast of the latest information about your disease.

Friends of ours moved to Arizona and swear that the climate makes their joints feel much better. Should we consider making a move like this?

Many people believe that packing up and moving to a warm, dry climate relieves the pain and stiffness of arthritis. While there's no evidence to prove this, a respite from shoveling snow in the cold winter months would no doubt make us all feel better. However, it's wise to consider all the variables before up-rooting yourself. Warm, dry weather may make you feel physically and emotionally better, but it cannot cure arthritis. In fact, for some people who have a good existing support system of friends and family, a move can prove to be a very isolating experience that may even be damaging to health. Make it a point to spend some time in any new location before deciding on a major move.

Can eliminating foods such as tomatoes and potatoes cure arthritis?

This is another popular myth. While eliminating foods from the nightshade family (which also includes eggplant and peppers) may help some people who have arthritis feel better, it does not constitute a cure.

How is arthritis diagnosed?

A medical history and thorough physical exami-nation are necessary in order to diagnose what type of arthritis you have. Your doctor needs to know which joints hurt, when they hurt, if pain is accom-panied by inflammation, and if you have injured or overused those joints in the past. Your doctor may ask you questions such as:

• Is the pain sharp or dull? How long does it last?

• Do you have pain on just one or on both sides of your body?

- Did the pain come on slowly? Or was it sudden?

- Is pain confined to certain joints or does it radiate to other parts of your body?

- At what time of day are your symptoms worst?

- What conditions make your symptoms worse? Do joints ache in damp weather? Are they aggravated by inactivity or exercise? Sitting or standing for long periods of time? Eating rich foods? Heat or cold?

- Do you have certain tender spots or points on your body?

- What kinds of foods do you eat?

- Do you exercise on a regular basis?

- Are you overweight?

- Are you under a great deal of stress? Have you recently experienced a major change in your life, such as a death in the family, dismissal from a job, or a move?

- What is your occupation? Do you perform repetitive movements in your work? Do you lift heavy objects?

- What sports do you play? Have you recently injured yourself or had operations due to injury in the past?

- Have you lost range of motion in your joints? For example, can you still raise your arms above your

head? Can you bend down to pick up the newspaper?

- Have you lost the ability to perform certain actions? Do you have trouble climbing the stairs or
buttoning your dress?

- Have you had other health problems in addition
to joint pain? Have you lost weight? Are you fe-
verish? Do you have any rashes on your skin?

- Has anyone else in your family experienced similar symptoms?

- Do you take any drugs? Drugs—legal and illegal,
prescription and over the counter—have side effects and interactions that may affect your condition. Be honest with your doctor about all drugs
that you take.

Are there any tests used to make a diagnosis of arthritis?

Yes. Your doctor may take a number of tests, including:

- Blood tests to measure factors such as hemoglobin
levels (which are low in cases of RA, lupus, and
ankylosing spondylitis), inflammation, rheumatoid
factor, enzymes, creatinine, and uric acid

- Urinalysis, which can indicate kidney damage due
to diseases such as lupus or scleroderma

- Imaging studies such as X rays, CAT (computed

axial tomography) scans, and MRIs (magnetic resonance imaging) to confirm a diagnosis and/or assess the extent of joint damage

- Joint aspiration, in which fluid from affected joints is drained and examined to determine factors such as the presence of crystals (as in gout) or cartilage fragments (as in OA)

- Biopsy, in which a small amount of tissue is removed and examined to detect evidence of systemic diseases such as lupus and scleroderma

- Arthroscopy, in which a doctor inserts a tiny tube into an affected joint for examination while you are under anesthesia

What health professionals might treat my arthritis?

The treatment of arthritis often involves a healthcare team that may consist of some of the following:

- Your family doctor is most likely an internist or general practitioner who had training in arthritis in medical school. When necessary, family doctors may refer you to a specialist.

- A rheumatologist is a specialist in arthritis and related diseases that affect the joints, bones, muscles, skin, and tissues.

- An orthopedic surgeon is a specialist in handling problems of the joints, bones, muscles, ligaments, and tendons. In addition to performing surgery, he or she may recommend braces, appropriate home care, or physical therapy.

- A physiatrist is a specialist in the design of comprehensive rehabilitation programs that might consist of physical therapy, regular exercise, and hot and cold packs.

- Podiatrists are specialists who treat arthritis in the feet.

- Pediatricians treat children who suffer from juvenile arthritis.

- An ophthalmologist is a specialist who provides eye care. (In the arthritis-related autoimmune disorder called Sjögren's syndrome, glands that produce tears become inflamed, resulting in red, itchy, or painful eyes.)

- A psychiatrist is a medical doctor who can help you deal with the emotional issues associated with coping with a chronic disease.

- A physical therapist is a medical professional who can teach you how to correctly perform exercises to achieve greater strength and flexibility. Physical therapists use a variety of techniques ranging from exercise and ultrasound to massage and electrical stimulation to strengthen your muscles and prevent your joints from growing stiff.

- An occupational therapist is a medical professional who can teach you how to sit, stand, lift, and move around without placing undue stress and strain on your joints. Occupational therapists can also fit you with splints, braces, and other supportive devices designed to protect your joints.

- Orthotists are specialists who design and fit orthotic devices (such as braces and splints) to help reduce pain and inflammation by stabilizing weak or damaged joints.

- Psychologists, who have Ph.D.s rather than M.D.s, can counsel you in coping with the mental and emotional issues associated with arthritis. Unlike psychiatrists, psychologists are not medical doctors and cannot prescribe medication.

- Social workers can help you cope with the social and financial challenges posed by arthritis.

What are the economic costs of arthritis?

Arthritis is estimated to cost the United States economy an enormous $65 billion each year in medical care and lost wages. Annual costs for hospitalizations from serious side effects of NSAID use are over $1 billion. Arthritis and musculoskeletal disorders are among the most common chronic health problems and are the leading cause of disability for Americans over the age of 65.

What are the social costs of arthritis? Will arthritis significantly interfere with my day-to-day life?

This depends on the type of arthritis you have and the severity of your condition. Minor symptoms will interfere little with day-to-day activities. Yet even in mild cases of arthritis, some adjustments are necessary. You must keep a sharper eye on your health from now on, watching diet and exercise and in many cases remembering to take medicine on a regular basis.

Severe arthritis can lead to much more significant changes in your daily life. Stiff and painful joints may make it increasingly difficult for you to get around and perform your normal activities. Simple tasks such as climbing the stairs, stooping down to pick up the newspaper, opening a can, or putting away the groceries may grow difficult and sometimes even impossible for arthritis sufferers. Your relationships with coworkers, friends, and family may be affected by your condition.

What is the emotional impact of arthritis?

Many people feel a sense of shock and disbelief when they first learn that they have a chronic disease. It's only natural to ask "Why me?" These initial feelings may be followed by anger and sadness before you come around to accepting your condition and coping with it in a positive way. Try to keep in mind that these emotions are only natural when you are dealing with major physical and emotional changes in your life.

How can my family and friends help?

It's important to harness the support of your friends and family in coping with arthritis. They cannot always tell when you are experiencing pain, and may at first resent or misunderstand your new limitations. Try to be open and honest about the physical changes taking place in your body and also your feelings about them.

Beyond friends and family, where else can I turn for help?

Many people join support groups for the social and emotional sustenance they gain from others who have the same disease. Some seek counseling from a psychiatrist, psychologist, or social worker. Your local branch of the Arthritis Foundation can provide a wealth of referrals, from medical doctors such as rheumatologists to special exercise classes for those who have arthritis.

What steps can I take to prevent arthritis from taking over my life?

In this book you will learn about many valuable strategies to manage your arthritis. They include exercise, diet, relaxation, stress control, and joint protection. Regular medication is very important, and remember that if you experience side effects such as ulcers and stomach bleeding due to nonsteroidal anti-inflammatory drugs, COX-2 inhibitors are a new alternative that may be right for you.

TWO

✦✦✦

What Kind of Arthritis Do You Have?

I live on the second floor, and the pain and swelling in my left knee used to make it hard to climb the stairs. I'd have to pause for a minute or two to make it all the way up. But it's better now. I just keep right on climbing until I get to the top.

Shirley Johnson, 53-year-old osteoarthritis patient
and participant in Celebrex clinical trials

Joint pain is the most common symptom linking the more than 100 different types of arthritis and related conditions. Increasing stiffness in your fingers, low back pain, swollen knees that making walking up the stairs seem more like climbing Mount Everest—these can all be the signs of arthritis.

Is there a cure for arthritis?

No, but there *are* many ways to manage your symptoms and slow the debilitating progress of this disease.

How is arthritis best managed?

Physical or occupational therapy and exercise enable you to retain and in some cases even increase your range of motion, while relaxation techniques can help you manage some of the pain, frustration, and emotional distress that too often accompany chronic diseases like arthritis. Weight control is important, and so is joint protection and learning everything you can about your disease. To that end, many people find joining support groups via the Arthritis Foundation beneficial.

But perhaps most importantly, medication can help you manage arthritis. A wide variety of anti-arthritis medications is available, and newer and more effective drugs are always in the pipeline. For example, NSAIDs (nonsteroidal anti-inflammatory drugs) have traditionally been used to control the pain and inflammation of arthritis. Unfortunately, NSAIDs can lead to gastrointestinal problems such as stomach bleeding and ulcers. In response, scientists have developed new medications called COX-2 inhibitors, that are as effective in controlling pain and inflammation as NSAIDs but in therapeutic doses are less likely to cause stomach-damaging side effects.

How can I tell what type of arthritis I have?

If you suffer from joint pain, it's important to see your doctor. Only a physician can correctly determine what type of arthritis you have and prescribe appropriate treatment. In order to do this, your doctor will take a careful medical history and examine you thoroughly, measuring your range of motion and checking for other clues such as inflammation, rashes, and tender points. Tests such as blood counts, urinalysis, imaging studies, and joint aspiration can help determine a diagnosis.

What is range of motion?

This is the extent to which you can move your arms, legs, or other parts of your body in any direction or at any angle. The stiff and painful joints of arthritis often limit your range of motion, or ROM. Strategies such as flexibility exercises can help you retain and sometimes even increase it.

Which forms of arthritis are COX-2 inhibitors prescribed for?

The FDA has so far approved COX-2 inhibitors for the treatment of osteoarthritis (both Celebrex and Vioxx) and rheumatoid arthritis (Celebrex alone). Since COX-2 inhibitors can effectively manage pain and inflammation with a significantly reduced incidence of gastrointestinal (GI) side effects, it is possible that in time these drugs will be prescribed for a wider variety of arthritic conditions.

What are some of the more common forms of arthritis and related conditions?

Osteoarthritis, the result of years of wear and tear on the joints, is the most common form of arthritis. Rheumatoid arthritis is another frequent problem, as are lupus, gout, fibromyalgia, and osteoporosis. In this chapter we examine the following forms of arthritis and related conditions:

- Osteoarthritis
- Rheumatoid arthritis
- Low back pain
- Bursitis and tendinitis
- Fibromyalgia syndrome
- Gout
- Systemic lupus erythematosus
- Lyme disease
- Osteoporosis
- Paget's disease
- Scleroderma
- Spondylitis

OSTEOARTHRITIS

More than 21 million Americans suffer from osteoarthritis (OA), which is by far the most common type of joint disease. Also known as degenerative arthritis, degenerative joint disease, or osteoarthrosis, this painful disorder is due to a gradual breakdown of joint cartilage and bones as we grow older. When cartilage covering the ends of the bones in a joint deteriorates, pain and loss of movement result. Heredity, injuries, overuse, and obesity can all contribute to the development of OA.

Who develops OA?

Osteoarthritis affects both men and women in the middle to later years. Up to the age of 45, osteoarthritis is more common in men than women. After age 45, it is more common in women.

What are the symptoms of osteoarthritis?

Osteoarthritis is a slowly developing disease that most commonly leads to pain and stiffness in the hips, knees, and spine. In this type of arthritis, joints tend to ache most if you overdo activity or move them after long periods of inactivity.

What are the causes of OA?

The breakdown of cartilage cushioning between the joints eventually leads to the pain and stiffness of osteoarthritis. Simple wear and tear is the most common cause.

What happens to the cartilage of OA sufferers?

Tough elastic tissue called cartilage normally covers the end of each bone in healthy joints, cushioning and supporting them. This smooth cartilage permits easy joint motion and acts as a shock absorber between the bones. But over the years, your cartilage gradually softens and becomes less elastic, which makes it more susceptible to wear-and-tear damage.

If I suspect that OA is my problem, when should I see my doctor?

The sooner, the better. Early intervention and treatment are best, for when degeneration is allowed to progress untreated, it becomes increasingly difficult to repair damaged cartilage.

What parts of the body are most commonly affected by OA?

Joints in the hips, knees, and back grow increasingly painful and stiff as the condition of cartilage deteriorates.

In addition to wear and tear, are there any other contributing factors to OA?

Injury and overuse of the joints also can lead to osteoarthritis:

- Athletes such as tennis, basketball, or football players often have knee injuries and operations to remedy them, which put them at greater risk for osteoarthritis in later years.

- Overuse of the same joints again and again is another risk factor for this disease. Studies show that miners and dockyard workers who perform repetitive motions suffer from higher rates of osteoarthritis than the rest of us.

Does OA run in families?

Yes. If your mother or grandmother suffered from backaches and swollen knees as she grew older, you too may develop these problems. In addition, if like other family members you tend to be overweight, the extra pounds you carry around make you more susceptible to developing osteoarthritis in the weight-bearing joints, which include your knees, feet, hips, and back.

I've put on a few pounds in the last few years. Does this increase my risk of developing OA?

It certainly does. While it's common to gain weight as the metabolism slows and we grow less active in middle age, be aware that the extra pounds you acquire put you at greater risk of developing OA and other health problems (such as high blood pressure and cardiovascular disease). Try to consume fewer calories and exercise more as you grow older in order to prevent excess pounds from accumulating around your middle.

To avoid pain and stiffness, I've cut back on my activities. Often I try to just sit still to keep the pain at bay. Is this a helpful strategy?

Unfortunately, no. Many people's instinctive response to stiffness and pain is to keep still—but this is exactly what you should *not* do, for a lack of exercise will only worsen your situation in the long run. Over time inactivity can cause the muscles surrounding a joint to weaken and even shrink. Weakened muscles provide less support for affected joints, leading to more pain when you eventually have to use them. If you have arthritis in your hip, for example, you may be tempted to spare yourself discomfort by sitting quietly and reading or watching TV instead of walking or swimming. But when you get out of bed in the morning, prepare a meal, or walk to the corner mailbox, you will find your hip stiffer and more achy than ever. Consult your doctor or physical therapist about a gentle, safe exercise program to keep your joints, muscles, and bones healthy.

How is osteoarthritis diagnosed?

A medical history and thorough physical examination are necessary in order to make the diagnosis. In addition, your doctor may take X rays, draw blood, or drain and examine some of the fluid from affected joints in a procedure called joint aspiration.

What medications are used to treat osteoarthritis?

A number of medications are prescribed to relieve the pain of OA as well as the swelling that occurs in some cases. They include:

• Analgesics to relieve pain

- In acute cases, even more powerful narcotic analgesics to relieve severe pain

- NSAIDs to relieve pain, stiffness, and inflammation

- New COX-2 inhibitors, such as Celebrex and Vioxx, which may be especially helpful alternatives when nonselective NSAIDs cause gastrointestinal side effects

- Corticosteroid injections to relieve pain and swelling

- Local pain-relieving creams and rubs to apply directly to the skin over a painful joint

How effective are COX-2 inhibitors in the treatment of OA?

In clinical studies, Celebrex significantly reduced the joint pain and stiffness of arthritis sufferers. The abilities of patients to walk, bend, and get in and out of cars improved. Celebrex's effectiveness was comparable to that of NSAIDs such as naproxen, while causing fewer GI side effects.

What is the recommended dosage of Celebrex for OA?

The recommended therapeutic dose is 200 milligrams daily, taken as a single dose or 100 milligrams twice a day. If you're like most people, you'll probably find it more convenient to take medication just once a day.

What other treatments are recommended for OA?

A variety of additional approaches are recommended for OA treatment. Exercise, heat and cold, joint protection, pacing activities, and self-care skills are all helpful. Weight control via diet and exercise is often recommended, and your doctor may also prescribe physical and/or occupational therapy. In very severe cases of osteoarthritis, surgery may be necessary.

RHEUMATOID ARTHRITIS

Rheumatoid arthritis (RA) is an autoimmune disease in which the linings of the joints become inflamed due to excessive immune system activity. Ordinarily the immune system is programmed to protect you from outside invaders such as viruses and bacteria. But in autoimmune diseases, a defect causes the body's immune system to turn on itself instead.

Potentially far more damaging than osteoarthritis, rheumatoid arthritis is fortunately also less common. Some 2 million Americans suffer the pain and inflammation of this very serious disease, which can affect joints in the hands, wrists, elbows, shoulders, feet, knees, and ankles on both sides of the body. Pain, disfigurement, and limited range of motion can occur in affected joints. Other organs too can be targeted as the disease progresses.

Who gets rheumatoid arthritis?

Rheumatoid arthritis is far more common in women than men. It usually affects young women between the ages of 25 and 50.

What are the symptoms of rheumatoid arthritis?

RA is often preceded by fatigue, fever, and weakness. Inflammation, pain, stiffness, and—in very severe cases—eventual destruction of the joints are typical. While the inflammation of rheumatoid arthritis begins in the linings of the joints, it may gradually progress until it damages cartilage, bone, and even organs such as the spleen, heart, or lungs.

What happens to joints in RA?

The inflamed joints of rheumatoid arthritis are red, warm, swollen, tender, and painful. These are due to inflammation of the synovium, or lining, of the joints. Immune system cells enter the synovium and aggravate the inflammation, leading to tissue damage. If you don't seek treatment, or in cases where the disease fails to respond to treatment, destruction of the joints, cartilage, bone, tendons, and ligaments may result, culminating in eventual joint deformity and disability.

What is the cause of rheumatoid arthritis?

Rheumatoid arthritis is an autoimmune disease of unknown origin. If you are susceptible to RA, the disease may be triggered by an infectious agent such as a virus.

How is rheumatoid arthritis diagnosed?

In a physical exam, your doctor may look for nodules (lumps that develop under the skin) at spots such as the back of your elbows. In addition to a thorough medical history and physical examination, your doctor may take X rays or other imaging studies of affected joints. Blood tests are also instrumental in diagnosing RA.

How are blood tests useful in diagnosing RA?

Although blood tests can offer no conclusive evidence of RA, they provide some very revealing information:

• An abnormal antibody called rheumatoid factor (RF) is present in the blood of more than three quarters of those who have RA.

• A low level of hemoglobin or red blood cells is a sign of a special type of anemia resulting from the chronic inflammation of RA. This result is also found in other types of arthritis—notably lupus, ankylosing spondylitis, psoriatic arthritis, and Reiter's syndrome—but not in OA.

- The erythrocyte sedimentation rate—or ESR or sed rate—can also be measured in a blood test. A high ESR indicates a high degree of inflammation, which can mean you have rheumatoid arthritis. In cases of OA (which usually does not involve inflammation), there is commonly a low ESR.

I've heard that pregnant women who have RA can develop carpal tunnel syndrome. Is this true?

Yes. Water retention can constrict the nerves in your wrists, leading to numbness in the fingers. While any pregnant woman can develop this condition, women who have rheumatoid arthritis seem to be more prone to it.

What are remissions and flares?

Rheumatoid arthritis is not uniformly painful. You may experience periods of remission, in which symptoms recede and you feel much better. At other times there will be flares, when pain, stiffness, and inflammation are at their worst. Regular rest is especially important at these times.

If my arthritis is in remission, can I stop taking my medication?

Absolutely not. In fact, it is often medication that sparks a remission. You should always take medication exactly as prescribed by your doctor. Do not skip doses or stop taking medication because you are feeling better.

What medications are used to treat rheumatoid arthritis?

Until recent years, RA—at least in its early stages—was treated primarily with NSAIDs to relieve pain and inflammation. Today stronger medications called DMARDs (disease-modifying antirheumatic drugs) are more aggressively prescribed at an earlier point to halt the progression of this very serious disease. DMARDs help manage immune system activity.

Are COX-2 inhibitors recommended for the treatment of RA?

Yes. For rheumatoid arthritis sufferers, the recommended dosage of Celebrex is 100 to 200 milligrams twice daily.

What about juvenile RA? Are COX-2 inhibitors ever prescribed for this problem?

Not yet, but this may happen very soon. G.D. Searle, the company that manufactures Celebrex, is currently working with the FDA to make this drug available to children who suffer from juvenile RA.

When are COX-2 inhibitors a good choice for RA sufferers?

If you have experienced GI problems such as diarrhea and stomach bleeding due to NSAIDs, ask your doctor about COX-2 inhibitors. These new drugs can control RA pain and inflammation as effectively as other NSAIDs, but may be a safer alternative as they are associated with fewer stomach problems.

What other treatments are recommended for rheumatoid arthritis?

Exercise, heat and cold, pacing activities, joint protection, and self-care are also emphasized in treatment. In very severe cases, surgery can be necessary.

When is surgery necessary?

When severe joint damage leads to extreme pain and disability, a total joint replacement may be necessary. In this procedure, an orthopedic surgeon will replace damaged parts of joints with metal and plastic components. Fortunately, total hip and total knee replacements have become relatively common and can help you remain independent.

What are the differences between osteoarthritis and rheumatoid arthritis?

There are a number of important differences:

- RA usually affects joints on both sides of the body, while OA (at least in its initial stages) affects the joints on only one side.

- RA often affects the small joints of the hands and feet, as well as the elbows, shoulders, and ankles;

OA most commonly affects the hips, knees, and back, and only rarely the elbows, shoulders, and ankles.

- RA usually affects women between 25 and 50, while OA affects both women and men from middle age onward.

- RA may come on suddenly, while OA takes years to develop.

- Unlike OA, RA causes swelling, redness, and warmth of joints.

- Unlike OA, RA causes overall weakness and fatigue, and is often accompanied by weight loss and fever.

LOW BACK PAIN

When most of us complain about our aching backs, we mean low back pain. Low back pain is a major cause of disability in the United States and other industrialized countries around the world. Interestingly, this problem is not nearly as common in less developed countries where people exercise more, eat fewer fatty foods, and have fewer weight problems.

Who gets low back pain?

At some point in our lives 8 out of 10 of us will find ourselves sidelined with low back pain. Back problems are influenced by heredity, lifestyle, and occupation:

- If your mother or father had a back problem, you are more likely to develop one too.

- Sitting for long periods of time and lifting heavy items on a regular basis are both notoriously tough on the back. If your job involves a lot of sitting or lifting—for example, if you drive a truck, sit at a computer, or lift heavy packages at a warehouse all day—you are more apt to have problems with your back.

- Other risk factors for low back pain include smoking, obesity, and stress.

What does smoking have to do with low back pain?

Smoking reduces the flow of oxygen-rich blood to the back.

What are the symptoms of low back pain?

Back pain can be sharp or dull, constant or intermittent. One type of very severe back pain is called sciatica.

What is sciatica?

This is one of the most vexing types of low back pain. Sciatica occurs when back problems irritate one or both of the large sciatic nerves that extend down from the back to each leg, causing sharp or burning pain to radiate down the buttocks to the legs. Sciatica is extremely painful, and can be accompanied by weakness, numbness, and an uncomfortable pins-and-needles kind of tingling sensation. In some cases, these sensations extend all the way to the feet.

What is the cause of low back pain?

Low back pain can be the result of injuries such as strains and sprains, or it may be due to arthritis. The lower or lumbar part of your back is constantly subjected to a very large load—the weight of your body—which puts it under great stress. Even a minor problem with the muscles, bones, ligaments, or tendons in the lumbar area may cause pain.

When should I suspect that low back pain is due to arthritis?

Chronic low back pain which lasts for longer than 12 weeks may be due to arthritis.

What are the risk factors for low back pain?

There are hundreds of things that can cause back pain. Some of the most common risk factors include:

• Being 30 to 60 years of age

• Sedentary occupation or lifestyle

- Long-distance driving

- Repeated bending or twisting

- Heavy lifting

- Participation in sports such as gymnastics, golf, diving, weight lifting, tennis, or football

- Obesity

- Depression, stress, or anxiety

- Dissatisfaction with work

- Smoking

- Poor posture

How is low back pain diagnosed?

Low back pain is notoriously difficult to diagnose; doctors are able to make the call in fewer than one in every five cases. But while it is not possible to determine the exact cause of each and every back problem, the good news is that we can effectively manage low back pain even when we don't know exactly what caused it.

How is low back pain treated?

Treatment is usually with NSAIDs to relieve pain and inflammation. Exercise, heat and cold, pacing of activities, joint protection, and self-care skills can also play invaluable roles in treatment.

Are COX-2 inhibitors ever used in the treatment of low back pain?

Vioxx has been approved for the treatment of acute general pain. G.D. Searle is also currently actively investigating the impact of Celebrex on this problem. If you experience gastrointestinal upset due to NSAIDs you are taking for back pain, ask your doctor whether COX-2 inhibitors may be an appropriate medication for you.

BURSITIS AND TENDINITIS

Nagging pains when you shoot a few baskets with your child or hunker down to work on your computer are sometimes due to bursitis or tendinitis. Bursitis affects small sacs called bursa which help muscles operate efficiently and easily, while tendinitis impacts the tendons that attach your muscles to your bones.

Who gets bursitis and tendinitis?

As we get older, injury and overuse make us more prone to developing bursitis and tendinitis.

What are the symptoms of bursitis and tendinitis?

The symptoms are pain and inflammation in affected areas. For example, if you work at a computer all day you might develop bursitis in your shoulder. Athletes such as basketball players may develop tendinitis in a knee, while tennis players nurse their "tennis elbows."

What are the causes of bursitis and tendinitis?

These conditions are the result of irritation due to injury or overuse of a joint.

How are bursitis and tendinitis diagnosed?

Your doctor will diagnose these problems after taking your medical history and conducting a careful physical examination.

How are bursitis and tendinitis treated?

Treatments include pain relievers and anti-inflammatory drugs, ice packs, heat, and rest.

Are COX-2 inhibitors ever prescribed to treat bursitis and tendinitis?

Vioxx has been approved to treat acute general pain. If you experience gastrointestinal upset due to medications, ask your doctor about COX-2 inhibitors. They may turn out to be an appropriate medication for you.

FIBROMYALGIA SYNDROME

Fibromyalgia is a chronic condition of muscle, tendon and ligament pain, disturbed sleep patterns, and relentless fatigue. Feelings of depression often accompany this vexing problem, which often defies both diagnosis and treatment. Fibromyalgia is much more common in women than in men, and is considered a syndrome rather than a disease.

Who gets fibromyalgia?

Fibromyalgia most frequently occurs in women between the ages of 20 and 50. It may affect as many as 2% of Americans.

What are the symptoms of fibromyalgia?

Widespread pain, tender points on the body, stiffness, disturbed sleep, and fatigue are all symptoms of this syndrome. Depression too often accompanies fibromyalgia, possibly due to either the frustrating symptoms themselves or because of the fact that this syndrome is so difficult to diagnose and treat.

What is the cause of fibromyalgia?

There are a number of theories, but at this point no one really knows for sure. Physical or emotional stresses may play a role in causing fibromyalgia in the first place or in triggering an attack. Some researchers believe that fibromyalgia is caused by small traumas to the muscles, due to a decrease in blood flow after an attack of the flu, an accident, or an emotional trauma. On the other hand, it may be that a sleep disorder is responsible. Interestingly, studies show that even very healthy people show symptoms of fibromyalgia when deprived of deep sleep.

My friends are frustrated with me and tell me nothing is really wrong. Are they right?

No. It's bad enough that fibromyalgia can be extremely debilitating and place significant limitations on your activities. It only makes matters worse when friends, family, or even doctors assume that you are making up your symptoms in order to gain attention or escape obligations. Be sure to set them straight.

How is fibromyalgia diagnosed?

Because its symptoms are suggestive of so many other disorders (such as chronic fatigue syndrome, silicone-associated rheumatic disease from breast implants, multiple chemical sensitivities, carpal tunnel syndrome, and multiple sclerosis), this syndrome is very difficult to diagnose. As of now there is no definitive laboratory test or X ray for fibromyalgia. Instead, the diagnosis is made when widespread pain and fatigue are present, and there are tender points at specific locations on the body.

How is fibromyalgia treated?

Patients are treated with medications that help them relax tense muscles and get a good night's sleep (most especially the important hours of deep, restorative sleep). Low doses of antidepressants, tranquilizers, and muscle relaxants are all helpful in this regard. Your doctor may also recommend an exercise program to increase your stamina and suggest that you practice relaxation techniques to relieve muscle tension, pain, and stress. Because of the peculiarly frustrating nature of this disease, many women find it helpful to attend support groups and educational classes about fibromyalgia.

Are COX-2 inhibitors ever prescribed for the treatment of fibromyalgia?

Not as of this point. NSAIDs do not have any major impact on this problem.

GOUT

Gout, a very common form of arthritis, is one of the oldest diseases in the world. It is the third most frequently seen type of arthritis, following OA and RA, but the easiest to diagnose and treat. Since an attack can be brought on by an overindulgence in food or wine, gout was once said to be "the rich man's disease." In fact, however, anyone who has trouble processing uric acid can fall victim to this painful affliction.

Who gets gout?

Gout is most common in men, often beginning around middle age. It may affect as many as 2% of Americans.

What are the symptoms of gout?

Gout usually affects only one joint at a time, and most often this is the big toe. Pain and swelling around the joint may develop after eating too much or drinking too much alcohol, or following a stressful event. Other joints that may be affected include the ankle, knee, foot, hand, wrist, or elbow.

What is the cause of gout?

Gout is the result of high uric acid levels in the body. These can be due either to excess production of uric acid or to an inability to excrete a sufficient amount of this waste product. Normally, after circulating through the blood, uric acid passes through the kidneys and out of the body as urine. When excess uric acid instead accumulates and solidifies, it forms into very painful, needlelike crystals that accumulate around extremities such as the big toe.

I've put on quite a bit of weight in my middle age. Does this put me at any extra risk of developing gout?

Yes. Being overweight and having high blood pressure (which often go hand in hand) are two risk factors for gout.

How is gout diagnosed?

Gout is a very easy disease to diagnose. A simple blood test reveals the telltale levels of uric acid, while fluid drawn from the affected joint indicates the presence of crystals.

How is gout treated?

Very effective medical treatment is available, including NSAIDs and drugs that specifically target gout. Diet is also important, and your doctor will suggest that you limit your alcohol intake and control your weight.

Are COX-2 inhibitors used in the treatment of gout?

Vioxx can be used to treat the acute general pain of gout. If you are taking NSAIDs for gout and consequently experience gastrointestinal upsets, ask your doctor whether Vioxx may be appropriate for you.

Are there any specific strategies I should follow in controlling gout?

Uric acid is the waste product of purines, which are compounds found in many foods. These include organ meats and fish such as sardines, herring, and mussels. Ask your doctor for a list of foods high in purines and try to eat them only in moderation.

SYSTEMIC LUPUS ERYTHEMATOSUS

Systemic lupus erythematosus—better known as simply lupus or SLE—is a potentially very serious rheumatic disease that affects the joints, organs, and skin. Like rheumatoid arthritis, lupus is an autoimmune disease due to a malfunctioning in the body's immune system. Eventually it may result in dangerous swelling of the lining of the heart, lungs, kidneys, nervous system, or abdomen. Fortunately, in recent years lupus has come to be managed more and more efficiently.

Who gets lupus?

Lupus is most common in women during the childbearing years. It tends to run in families, and is more common among African Americans, Latinos, Native Americans, and Asians.

What are the symptoms of lupus?

Most common are arthralgia (achy joints), a fever over 100 degrees Fahrenheit (38 degrees Centigrade), the swollen joints of arthritis, prolonged fatigue, and skin rashes. A butterfly-shaped rash across the cheeks and nose is one of the most classic signs of lupus, but this actually occurs in a little less than half of all cases. Rashes may also develop elsewhere on the body, and are often brought on by exposure to the sun. Other signs of lupus are:

- Anemia

- Kidney involvement

- Pleurisy (pain in the chest when you breathe deeply that is unrelated to position or movement)

- Rash, hives, and skin sores

- Photosensitivity

- Hair loss

- Raynaud's phenomenon (fingers turn white and/or blue in the cold)

- Seizures

- Mouth ulcers

Are the symptoms of lupus always the same?

No. Most people who have lupus do not have all these symptoms. In addition, lupus follows a similar pattern to rheumatoid arthritis in terms of remission and flares. At times you will experience flares, when symptoms are at their worst. Regular rest is necessary at these times. You may also have periods of remission in which symptoms fade and you feel much better. Take these opportunities to exercise more for joint flexibility and muscle strength.

What is the cause of lupus?

Lupus is an autoimmune disease of unknown origin. Hormonal and genetic factors are thought to play a role in this disease, which occurs 10 times more frequently in women than in men. Estrogen is probably a factor, since pregnancy and birth control use stimulate increased lupus activity. If you are susceptible to lupus, it may be triggered by environmental factors such as ultraviolet rays, which cause sunburn, or the use of certain drugs.

How is lupus diagnosed?

It is often difficult to diagnose lupus because symptoms vary and may masquerade as those of other diseases. If your doctor suspects that you have lupus, you will undergo a blood test to detect the presence of specific antinuclear antibodies associated with this disease. Excess protein in the urine, a low white blood cell count, or low platelet count too are symptoms of SLE. Kidney function tests may also be performed.

What medications are used to treat lupus?

This depends on your particular case. NSAIDs are usually prescribed to deal with pain, stiffness, and inflammation. If skin rashes are a problem, topical cortisone creams are useful. When these don't do the trick, your doctor may prescribe prednisone to be taken orally. Higher doses of prednisone are necessary if lupus is causing inflammation of the lining of the heart or lungs, or if your platelet count is low. DMARDs, more powerful than NSAIDs, are prescribed in certain cases to control immune system activity.

Are COX-2 inhibitors ever prescribed for the treatment of lupus?

Vioxx can be used to relieve acute general pain. Therefore if NSAIDs that you are taking for the relief of lupus symptoms are causing you gastrointestinal distress, ask your doctor about Vioxx.

What other treatments are recommended for lupus?

Self-care is important. You must watch your diet, and make sure that you get a good balance of rest and exercise. Many people find it helpful to join support groups via the Arthritis Foundation or the Lupus Foundation.

LYME DISEASE

Lyme disease is a form of infectious arthritis. After being bitten by a tiny deer tick, a rash and flulike symptoms may be followed by arthritis in the hips, knees, shoulders, and other joints.

What are the symptoms of Lyme disease?

Three to 30 days after being bitten by an infected tick, a telltale bull's-eye rash usually (but not always) develops around the bite. Flulike symptoms such as a fever, severe headache, aching muscles and joints, and swollen glands occur, and may later be followed by the pain and stiffness of arthritis. The heart and nervous system can be affected.

What is the cause of Lyme disease?

Lyme disease is a bacterial infection spread by a deer tick the size of the head of a pin.

How is Lyme disease diagnosed?

Lyme disease often mimics the symptoms of other disorders, and even the telltale bull's-eye rash does not occur in all cases. However, doctors have now developed a test to determine if Lyme disease is the problem.

How is Lyme disease treated?

When Lyme disease is diagnosed at an early point, it can be promptly and successfully treated with antibiotics. In some cases, your doctor may prescribe or recommend NSAIDs to manage pain and inflammation. Unfortunately, chronic Lyme arthritis may develop in a small number of susceptible individuals.

Do COX-2 inhibitors have any role in the treatment of Lyme disease?

COX-2 inhibitors are not approved to treat Lyme disease. However, if you experience gastrointestinal upset due to NSAIDs, ask your doctor about them.

OSTEOPOROSIS

Osteoporosis, which causes the bones to become thin and brittle, is a silent, progressively more dangerous arthritis-related disease. Many women don't even realize that they have osteoporosis until they suddenly break a hip or wrist, or experience the painful collapse of a fragile vertebra.

Who gets osteoporosis?

Medical experts estimate that more than 24 million Americans suffer from this bone-thinning disease. At greatest risk are postmenopausal women of northern European or Asian descent. Other risk factors include:

- A family history of osteoporosis
- Fair skin
- Slight build
- Sedentary lifestyle
- Smoking
- Insufficient calcium intake
- Long-term use of corticosteroids
- Excessive alcohol consumption
- Early onset of menopause
- Eating disorders

What does osteoporosis have to do with menopause?

The process of bone deterioration rapidly accelerates in women when estrogen levels drop at menopause.

Don't men ever get osteoporosis?

Yes, although far less frequently than women. Men account for about 20 percent of osteoporosis cases.

How is osteoporosis diagnosed?

The bone densitometry test is one of the best diagnostic tools. As you approach menopause, get a realistic assessment of your risk by asking your doctor to measure your bone density. X rays alone cannot detect osteoporosis, because by the time an ordinary X ray detects a problem you may have already lost as much as 30 percent of your bone mass. Morcover, bone density tests are very safe and give off even less radiation than standard X rays.

My mother suffered terribly from osteoporosis, with one fracture after another. What can I do to keep from developing this disease myself? Are there any helpful steps I can recommend to my teenage daughter?

Fortunately, there are many things you can do to prevent osteoporosis. It is never too early to start taking measures to prevent this disease, nor is it ever too late to try to thwart it. Use these helpful strategies:

- **Drink your milk**. A calcium-rich diet strengthens bones and can help prevent osteoporosis. If you don't get enough of this important mineral in your regular diet, ask your doctor to prescribe a supplement.

- **Do regular weight-bearing exercises.** To strengthen your bones, squeeze in 20 to 30 minutes of walking, jogging, dancing, biking, or lifting free weights at least three times each week.

- **Consider hormone replacement therapy.** Hormones play a key role in maintaining strong, healthy bones, and for many menopausal women this means hormone replacement therapy or HRT. Others opt for natural hormone therapy, such as the application of natural progesterone cream or incorporating phytoestrogens into their diets. To determine whether or not it is right for you, discuss the benefits and risks of HRT with your doctor.

How much calcium is necessary to prevent bone loss?

Before menopause, try to include 1,200 milligrams of calcium and 400 international units of vitamin D in your diet each day. Vitamin D is necessary for the efficient absorption of calcium. When estrogen levels fall at menopause, increase your calcium intake to

1,500 milligrams a day. To get an idea of what these numbers mean, one 8-ounce glass of milk contains 300 milligrams of calcium.

At 65, I think I'm past the point of preventing osteoporosis. Is there any reason for me to try to fight it now?

Fortunately, it's never too late to start building bone mass. Even women who have already fractured a hip can strengthen their bones through regular, gentle exercise and a calcium-rich diet.

How is osteoporosis treated?

In addition to self-help measures, prescribed medications can help control osteoporosis. Estrogen in hormone replacement therapy offers protection against brittle bones, as do calcitonin (another hormone) and alendronate. Alendronate reduces the risk of vertebral fractures by almost half in postmenopausal women who have osteoporosis.

PAGET'S DISEASE

Paget's disease causes bones in the spine and elsewhere in the body to thicken and sometimes grow crumbly. This disease has been linked to a number of back ailments, including arthritis and vertebral compression fractures due to weakened bones.

Who gets Paget's disease?

Fortunately, this is not a very common disease. It most frequently strikes people over the age of 50.

What are the symptoms of Paget's disease?

Paget's disease produces excessive remodeling and overgrowth of bone, especially in the spine, pelvis, skull, and femur. In severe cases, bones in the spine can grow in to the spinal canal, where they press painfully on the spinal cord and nerves.

How is Paget's disease treated?

People who experience pinched nerves and back pain due to Paget's disease are treated with a number of medications. Calcitonin and alendronate, which are both used to treat osteoporosis, can be helpful in the treatment of Paget's disease. NSAIDs may be prescribed or recommended for local pain and inflammation.

Are COX-2 inhibitors ever prescribed for the treatment of Paget's disease?

It's possible. If you are taking NSAIDs for pain and inflammation and they cause you gastrointestinal distress, ask your doctor about Vioxx.

SCLERODERMA

This is a chronic, autoimmune disease of the connective tissue. Scleroderma, which literally means "hard skin," can cause the skin on the hands, arms, and face to grow thick and hard. But this is a highly variable problem and sometimes involves the connective tissue in other parts of the body, including the blood vessels, muscles, joints, esophagus, gastrointestinal tract, heart, lungs, and kidneys.

Who gets scleroderma?

This disease, which is also known as systemic sclerosis, most frequently affects women between the ages of 30 and 60.

What are the symptoms of scleroderma?

Scleroderma is noticeable when the skin is affected, but invisible when only the internal organs are involved. The symptoms range from mild to life-threatening. The first signs may be a frostbite-like bluish tint, tingling, and numbness in the fingers. Fingers turning pale or bluish upon exposure to the cold is called Raynaud's phenomenon. Muscles, joints, and organs may sustain damage due to overproduction of collagen.

What are the causes of scleroderma?

Its exact cause is unknown. Like rheumatoid arthritis and lupus, scleroderma is an autoimmune disease of unknown origin. It may be triggered by environmental factors.

How is scleroderma diagnosed?

Diagnosis is difficult, since the symptoms of scleroderma often mimic those of other autoimmune diseases. It may require blood tests, other tests depending on what organs are involved, and consultation with rheumatologists and dermatologists. Many cases of scleroderma may go undiagnosed.

How is scleroderma treated?

There is no cure for scleroderma, but treatment with drugs such as penicillamine and colchicine may be helpful.

SPONDYLITIS

Spondylitis—the most common type of which is ankylosing spondylitis or AS—is a painful type of arthritis that affects the joints of vertebrae in the back, causing them to become stiff and swollen. Spondylitis can also attack the joints of the extremities—the hips, shoulders, and knees—and nearby ligaments and tendons at the points where they attach to bones.

Who gets spondylitis?

This type of arthritis ordinarily runs in families, and most often strikes young men in their twenties and thirties.

What are the symptoms of spondylitis?

The low back pain and stiffness typical of this problem come on slowly and gradually worsen over time. Symptoms are worst in the mornings. As you become more active in the course of the day or take a hot shower, you'll feel better.

What is the cause of this disease?

Spondylitis is an autoimmune disease of unknown origin. It is usually hereditary.

How is spondylitis diagnosed?

As with other forms of arthritis, your doctor will examine you, obtain a careful medical history, and take X rays. One important clue to diagnosing spondylitis is its particular pattern of pain: Unlike many other forms of arthritis, relief comes with exercise, while bed rest worsens pain and discomfort. Your doctor will be careful to distinguish ankylosing spondylitis from Reiter's syndrome and psoriatic arthritis, two related conditions that involve similar inflammations of the spinal joints.

How is spondylitis treated?

NSAIDs are prescribed to relieve the pain and inflammation of spondylitis. At times DMARDs, or disease-modifying antirheumatic drugs, are also prescribed to help control immune system activity.

Exercise, heat and cold, pacing activities, joint protection, self-care skills, and support groups may all
play a part in treatment. In very severe cases, the vertebrae can become fused into a stiff rod, making
movement very difficult and painful. When deformi-
ties become this crippling, they must be corrected
with surgery.

Do COX-2 inhibitors have any role in the treatment of ankylosing spondylitis?

The Spring 1999 issue of *Spondylitis Plus*—the
quarterly publication of the Spondylitis Association of
America—features an article on the FDA approval of
the "long-awaited new class of NSAIDs with potential
for fewer gastrointestinal problems," led by the new
COX-2 inhibitor Celebrex.

Are the manufacturers of COX-2 inhibitors looking into their potential for treating spondylitis?

Vioxx has been approved for the treatment of acute
general pain. In addition, Searle is conducting an on-
going study in Europe to examine the role of Celebrex
in the treatment of spondylitis.

THREE

~~~~~

Standard Drug Therapy for Arthritis

*I feel 100 percent better since I've been taking Ce-
lebrex. With other medications, I had to watch everything I ate. If I took them on an empty stomach, I
threw up. Now my pain is gone and I can eat anything I want.*

Frank Edwards, 57-year-old osteoarthritis and
rheumatoid arthritis patient, and participant in
Celebrex clinical trials

Sooner or later almost everyone who suffers from arthritis turns to medication of one kind or another.
Some drugs are available over-the-counter (OTC),
while others are obtainable by prescription only.
Among the many anti-arthritis drugs available today
are corticosteroids, DMARDs, and topical analgesics,
as well as special medications for osteoporosis, fibromyalgia, and gout. However, the most widely used
drugs by far are NSAIDs like aspirin, ibuprofen, and
naproxen. These medications offer relief from the

pain and inflammation of arthritis, but over the years a troubling problem has been their sometimes serious side effects, including diarrhea, ulcers, and internal bleeding. Because they are equally effective yet reduce the incidence of these side effects, COX-2 inhibitors such as Celebrex and Vioxx have rapidly become an enormously attractive alternative to arthritis sufferers.

NSAIDs

What are NSAIDs?

Nonsteroidal anti-inflammatory drugs, or NSAIDs, are the most commonly used medications for arthritis. An arsenal of more than 20 different NSAIDs are taken today to help control the pain and inflammation of arthritis. Unfortunately, these drugs may also irritate the stomach lining and in some cases lead to gastrointestinal bleeding and ulcers.

What are some examples of NSAIDs?

Following is a list of the major NSAIDs for the treatment of arthritis. Salicylates—including aspirin, the oldest NSAID—are a subcategory of NSAIDs. Celebrex and Vioxx are the new COX-2 inhibitors, another subcategory of NSAIDs.

The drugs that follow are identified by their generic names followed by their brand names:

- Celecoxib (Celebrex)

- Diclofenac potassium (Cataflam)

- Diclofenac sodium (Voltaren)

- Etodalac (Lodine)

- Fenoprofen calcium (Nalfon)

- Flurbiprofen (Ansaid)

- Ibuprofen (prescription: Motrin; OTC: Motrin IB, Advil, Nuprin)

- Indomethacin (Indocin)

- Ketoprofen (prescription: Orudis, Oruvail; OTC: Actron, Orudis KT)

- Ketorolac (Toradol)

- Meclofenamate sodium (Meclomen)

- Mefenamic acid (Ponstel)

- Nabumetone (Relafen)

- Naproxcn (Naprosyn)

- Naproxen sodium (prescription: Anaprox; OTC: Aleve)

- Oxaprozin (Daypro)

- Piroxicam (Feldene)

- Sulindac (Clinoril)

- Tolmetin sodium (Tolectin)

- Salicylates
  Aspirin (Anacin, Bayer, Bufferin, Ecotrin, Excedrin)

Choline magnesium trisalicylate (CMT, Tricosal, Trilisate)

Choline salicylate (Arthropan)

Diflunisal (Dolobid)

Magnesium salicylate (Magan, Doan's Pills, Mobidin)

Salsalate (Amigesic, Anaflex 750, Disalcid, Marthritic, Mono-Gesic, Salflex, Salsitab)

Sodium salicylate (generic)

Are NSAIDs available by prescription or over-the-counter (OTC)?

For many years, aspirin was the only NSAID available on an over-the-counter basis. OTC refers to over-the-counter drugs for which you don't need a prescription. Today ibuprofen, naproxen sodium, and ketoprofen are also available OTC.

Are COX-2 inhibitors available by prescription or over the counter?

COX-2 inhibitors are available only by prescription from your doctor.

What are the possible side effects of NSAIDs?

There are many potential problems, which may be even worse if you have a pre-existing problem such as heart or kidney disease. They include:

• Abdominal cramps and pain

- Diarrhea

- Fluid retention

- Ulcers

- Gastrointestinal bleeding

- Heartburn

- Indigestion

- Nausea

- Vomiting

- Greater tendency to bruise or bleed from cuts

- Confusion

- Deafness

- Dizziness

- Drowsiness

- Lightheadedness

- Nightmares

- Ringing in the ears (tinnitus)

- Rash

Is there anyone who should *not* take NSAIDs?

Yes. Your doctor may instruct you not to take NSAIDs if:

- You are sensitive or allergic to aspirin

- You have kidney or liver disease

- You have heart disease or high blood pressure

- You have an ulcer

- You suffer from asthma

- You are taking blood thinners

How serious are the side effects of NSAIDs?

They can be extremely serious. A recent study estimated that complications of NSAID use including gastrointestinal bleeding and perforation led to 107,000 hospitalizations and 16,500 deaths in this country each year. New COX-2 inhibitors such as Celebrex and Vioxx were developed specifically to reduce the occurrence of these troubling side effects.

Is there anything I can do to lessen some of the side effects of NSAIDs?

Here are some helpful steps you can take:

- Alert your doctor promptly if you experience any gastrointestinal problems.

- Have regular checkups, because ulcers and internal bleeding can occur without your even knowing about them.

- To avoid stomach upset, take medication with meals (or at least along with a few crackers or a slice of bread), a glass of milk, or an antacid.

- Do not drink alcohol while taking NSAIDs. In addition to causing kidney and liver damage, alcohol can increase your risk of ulcers and stomach bleeding.

- To control diarrhea, avoid greasy or spicy foods and dairy products. Instead eat binding foods (for example, rice and bananas) and drink plenty of electrolyte-rich fluids (such as herbal teas, vegetable broths, and electrolyte-replacement drinks). A cup of plain yogurt or a lactobacillus acidophilus supplement can help restore the normal balance of intestinal bacteria.

- When stomach distress is a problem, ask your doctor to prescribe enteric-coated NSAIDs. Enteric-coated tablets are also easier to swallow.

- Your physician can prescribe nonacetylated salicylates (which include all the salicylates except aspirin), which are specially formulated to be easy on the stomach and kidneys.

- Ask about longer-acting NSAIDs such as diclofenac sodium, oxaprozin, controlled-release naproxen, and etodolac extended-relief. These pills may be easier on your stomach since they only have to be taken once a day.

- Your doctor may also prescribe or recommend drugs to prevent ulcers. These include cimetidine (Tagamet), ranitidine hydrochloride (Zantac), famotidine (Pepcid), nizatidine (Axid Pulvules), omeprazole (Prilosec), lansoprazole (Prevacid), and misoprostol (Cytotec).

- Ask your doctor about new COX-2 inhibitors, which are less likely to cause stomach problems than traditional NSAIDs.

Is it best to take NSAIDs *with* meals or *after* meals?

Take NSAIDs *with* meals.

Will taking NSAIDs for long periods cause physical damage?

This is an unfortunate possibility. Ulcers, stomach bleeding, and other gastrointestinal effects tend to be more common in long-term users.

How do COX-2 inhibitors compare to NSAIDs for long-term users? Will their long-term use cause stomach damage?

Not that we know of. But keep in mind that COX-2 inhibitors have only recently been approved by the FDA. While they seem to be a safer alternative, only time will tell for sure. And while COX-2 inhibitors do reduce the risk of gastrointestinal side effects, they cannot eliminate them altogether.

How will my doctor decide which NSAID is right for me?

Your doctor will examine you and decide on an appropriate NSAID based on the type, severity, and longevity of your symptoms. Each NSAID has a unique effect on your body, so it may take several tries with different drugs before your doctor finds the one that works best for you.

I've been taking NSAIDs for my arthritis for several years. Should I ask my doctor to change my prescription to a COX-2 inhibitor?

Not necessarily. Arthritis sufferers who have taken NSAIDs without encountering stomach problems should stay with them, according to the FDA. But if you experience ulcers, stomach bleeding, or other gastrointestinal problems as a result of taking traditional NSAIDs, you should be aware that COX-2 inhibitors cause fewer of these problems and may be a better alternative for you.

When should I take my medication?

For minor aches and pains, over-the-counter NSAIDs can be taken as needed. Just be sure to carefully follow the directions on the package. But when pain and inflammation are persistent or severe, your doctor will prescribe a more powerful NSAID. These medications are usually taken once or twice daily, as per your doctor's instructions, in the morning or evening at the same time each day. If you have OA, your doctor can prescribe a COX-2 inhibitor. For example, Celebrex must be taken either once or twice a day. If you have RA, you must take Celebrex twice a day. Vioxx, approved for the treatment of OA but not RA, is taken once daily.

How do NSAIDs work?

Scientists believe that NSAIDs work by blocking or inhibiting the cyclooxygenase (COX) enzymes that produce prostaglandins.

What are prostaglandins?

Prostaglandins are hormonelike chemicals in the body that make nerve endings more sensitive and intensify the pain and inflammation of arthritis.

What is the role of the COX enzymes in the body?

As it turns out there are two types of cyclooxygenase enzymes, which scientists have designated COX 1 and COX 2. COX 2 is responsible for the inflammation of arthritis, while COX 1 protects the stomach lining. Unfortunately, until now, all NSAIDs indiscriminately or nonselectively attacked both enzymes. In more selective COX-2 inhibitors such as Celebrex and Vioxx, the focus is on blocking only the COX 2 enzyme.

This is a little confusing. What is the difference between these two enzymes?

COX 1, nicknamed the "housekeeping" enzyme, protects your stomach lining. Blocking it—as aspirin, ibuprofen, and other conventional NSAIDs do—can lead to GI problems such as bleeding and ulcers.

COX 2 is the enzyme most closely associated with the pain and inflammation of arthritis. COX-2 inhibitors such as Celebrex and Vioxx block primarily the COX 2 enzyme, and thus cause fewer gastrointestinal side effects.

Why do NSAIDs upset the stomach?

Conventional NSAIDs inhibit or suppress enzymes that produce hormonelike chemicals called prostaglandins, which protect the stomach from its own erosive acids.

How do COX-2 inhibitors manage to control pain without, in most cases, bothering the stomach?

Therapeutic doses of COX-2 inhibitors move directly to the source of arthritis pain. There they suppress the enzymes that produce the prostaglandins that cause pain and swelling. In therapeutic doses they have little or no effect on the prostaglandins that protect your stomach, so these chemicals can go right on doing their job.

Does this mean that COX-2 inhibitors will eventually come to replace conventional NSAIDs?

Probably not. The FDA recommends that you keep taking your usual NSAIDs as long as they are not causing stomach problems. Many of these drugs (such as aspirin) have long and impressive safety records. Although the new COX-2 inhibitors appear very safe, it takes time for any new drug to prove itself and establish a safety record.

Does aspirin possess any advantages over COX-2 inhibitors?

Yes. Beyond its impressive and proven track record for safety, aspirin has a protective effect on your heart. Blood-thinning aspirin blocks COX 1, which is responsible for the blood clots that can eventually lead to heart disease. Dr. Philip Needham, a developer of the first FDA-approved COX-2 inhibitor, believes that someday we'll all be taking a baby aspirin a day to protect our hearts while reserving COX-2 inhibitors like Celebrex for relief of pain and inflammation of problems such as arthritis.

What happens if I can't tolerate the side effects of NSAIDs?

Other options such as COX-2 inhibitors are available. When pain alone is a problem, analgesics such as acetaminophen may be helpful.

ANALGESICS

What are analgesics?

Analgesics are drugs that relieve pain. Unlike NSAIDs, they do not have any impact on inflammation.

How are aspirin-free analgesics useful in the treatment of arthritis?

Aspirin-free pain relievers such as acetaminophen are a good alternative for people who have an ulcer, are allergic to aspirin, or cannot tolerate the gastrointestinal side effects of aspirin and other NSAIDs. They are primarily helpful in cases of osteoarthritis and other noninflammatory problems. Again, while analgesics provide pain relief, they have no impact on swelling and inflammation.

What are some examples of analgesics?

Following is a list of the major analgesics for the treatment of arthritis. Some analgesics also contain caffeine (to gain quicker pain relief), antihistamines (to make you drowsy when pain prevents you from getting a good night's sleep), or codeine (for very severe pain). Drugs are identified by their generic names followed by their brand names:

- Acetaminophen (Aspirin-Free Anacin, Excedrin Caplets, Panadol, Tylenol)

- Acetaminophen with Codeine (Fioricet, Phenaphen with Codeine, Tylenol with Codeine)

- Propoxyphene hydrochloride (Darvon, PC-Cap, Wygesic)

- Tramadol (Ultram)

Are analgesics available by prescription or over the counter?

It varies. Plain acetaminophen is available over the counter. Other drugs listed above are only available by prescription.

Do analgesics cause any side effects?

Yes. Even though acetaminophen and other analgesics cause fewer side effects than NSAIDs, their long-term use can harm the liver and kidneys. Narcotic pain relievers (those that contain codeine) are potentially addictive, and must be used with extreme care. For this reason, narcotics are usually recommended only on a short-term basis for controlling the acute pain of arthritis flares. Although it is not a narcotic, there is also a small risk of addiction with tramadol.

CORTICOSTEROIDS

What are corticosteroids?

Corticosteroids are medications that suppress dangerous inflammation in the body. The impact of these drugs—which are chemical reproductions of hormones naturally manufactured by the adrenal glands—is swift and significant. With their dramatic impact on rheumatoid arthritis, corticosteroids were considered to be virtual miracle drugs when they were first introduced earlier in the twentieth century. But this was before their severe side effects came to light.

Are corticosteroids available by prescription or over the counter?

Corticosteroids, with potentially very serious side effects, are powerful drugs that must be prescribed by your doctor. Your doctor will carefully monitor your health while you are taking them, as side effects include serious problems such as reducing your resistance to infection.

What are the possible side effects of corticosteroids?

There are many potential problems, including:

- Bloating and puffiness

- Increased appetite

- Weight gain

- Brittle bones

- Nervousness

- Insomnia

- Mood changes

- High blood pressure

- Cataracts

- Elevated blood sugar

What are some examples of corticosteroids?

Following is a list of the major corticosteroids for the treatment of arthritis. Drugs are identified by their generic names followed by their brand names:

- Cortisone (Cortone Acetate)

- Dexamethasone (Decadron, Hexadrol)

- Hydrocortisone (Cortef, Hydrocortone)

- Methylprednisolone (Medrol)

- Prednisolone (Prelone)

- Prednisolone sodium phosphate (Pediapred)

- Prednisone (Deltasone, Orasone, Prednicen-M, Sterapred)

- Triamcinolone (Aristocort)

Is there anyone who should *not* take corticosteroids?

Do not take corticosteroids if you have:

- A fungal infection

- Inactive tuberculosis

- An underactive thyroid

- Herpes simplex of the eye

- High blood pressure

- Osteoporosis

- An ulcer

What about glucocorticoids?

Prescribed to reduce even more severe pain and inflammation, injections of glucocorticoids can only be used a few times a year, as they may weaken bone, tendons, and cartilage.

DISEASE-MODIFYING ANTIRHEUMATIC DRUGS (DMARDs)

What are DMARDs?

Powerful disease-modifying antirheumatic drugs, or DMARDs, are prescribed to slow and in some cases even halt the destructive process of rheumatoid arthritis. Yet though the hope is that they prevent or reduce joint damage, DMARDs such as oral and injectable gold have significant side effects. In addition, they may take from several weeks to months to work.

Are DMARDs ever prescribed for any other types of arthritis?

Some DMARDs are also prescribed for other inflammatory diseases, including lupus, ankylosing spondylitis, and Sjögren's syndrome.

When are DMARDs prescribed?

The use of these drugs has traditionally been reserved to the most serious cases because the side effects of the various DMARDs are both extensive and serious. Yet in recent years doctors have taken a more aggressive stance against RA, using DMARDs early on to try to halt the relentless progression of this disease and prevent irreversible damage.

What are the possible side effects of DMARDs?

Side effects are potentially very serious, and vary widely from DMARD to DMARD. They range all the way from gastrointestinal problems, tremors, and bleeding gums to kidney and liver damage, infertility, and increased susceptibility to infection.

Whenever you take disease modifiers, it is very important that your doctor carefully monitor you for side effects. For example, you may be required to undergo blood and urine tests to make sure drugs are not harming your liver or kidneys.

How do DMARDs work?

Scientists don't know the answer to this question. Although they appear to modify the immune system in some way, just how DMARDs do this remains a mystery.

Are DMARDs available by prescription or over-the-counter?

DMARDs are very powerful drugs that are only available by prescription from your doctor. Your doctor will carefully monitor your health while you are taking DMARDs because among their many serious side effects is a tendency to reduce your resistance to infection.

What are some examples of DMARDs?

Following is a list of the major DMARDs for the treatment of arthritis. Drugs are identified by their generic names followed by their brand names:

- Auranofin (Gold)

- Azathioprine (Imuran)

- Cyclophosphamide (Cytoxan)

- Cyclosporine (Sandimmune)

- Hydroxychloroquine-sulfate (Plaquenil)

- Methotrexate (Rheumatrex)

- Minocycline (Minocin)

- Penicillamine (Cuprimine, Depen)

- Sulfasalazine (Azulifidine)

Is there anyone who should *not* take DMARDs?

There are many people who should not take DMARDs. Among the more common reasons to avoid these drugs are a history of kidney or liver disease, inflammatory bowel disease, blood disease, alcoholism, or high blood pressure. Just as the side effects vary according to the individual disease-modifying drug in question, so do cautions and contraindications. These are issues you must carefully explore with your physician.

FIBROMYALGIA MEDICATIONS

Do traditional anti-inflammatory medications have much of an impact on fibromyalgia?

Not really. Over-the-counter aspirin, acetaminophen, or ibuprofen may provide some pain relief, but they do not have any major impact on fibromyalgia.

Are there special medications for fibromyalgia?

Yes. Medications that relax muscles and promote deeper sleep, when carefully prescribed in low doses for bedtime use, help women with fibromyalgia get a much needed and often all too rare good night's sleep. Unfortunately, sleep aids are also potentially addictive.

What are some examples of fibromyalgia medications?

Following is a list of some of the major drugs for the treatment of fibromyalgia. Medications are identified by their generic names followed by their brand names:

- Tricyclic Antidepressants
    Amitriptyline hydrochloride (Elavil, Endep)
    Doxepin (Adapin, Sinequan)
    Nortriptyline (Aventyl, Pamelor)

- SSRIs (Selective Serotonin Reuptake Inhibitors)
    Fluoxetine (Prozac)
    Paroxetine (Paxil)
    Sertraline (Zoloft)

- Benzodiazepines
    Temazepam (Restoril)

- Muscle Relaxants
    Cyclobenzaprine (Cycloflex, Flexeril)

This is a little confusing. Why are antidepressants prescribed for arthritis sufferers?

Antidepressants are useful in relieving chronic pain, even in those who are not depressed. They work by influencing the hormone levels that control sleep and pain. They are more often prescribed in cases of fibromyalgia than in other types of arthritis.

Is there anyone who should not take fibromyalgia medications?

Like all medications, the antidepressants and muscle relaxants used in these cases have side effects. Likewise, their rate of improvement varies. Only your doctor can determine what medications are right for you.

GOUT MEDICATIONS

Are there special medications for gout?

Yes. Gout, a common and painful type of arthritis, is the result of excess uric acid in the body. Drugs that control the level of uric acid are therefore prescribed along with NSAIDs to control the symptoms of gout.

What are some examples of gout medications?

Following is a list of the major drugs for the treatment of gout. Medications are identified by their generic names followed by their brand names:

- Allopurinol (Lopurin, Zyloprim)

- Colchicine (generic)

- Probenecid and Colchicine (ColBENEMID, Proben-C)

- Probenecid (Benemid, Probalan)

- Sulfinpyrazone (Anturane)

How do gout medications work?

Allopurinol helps control excess production of uric acid, while probenecid and sulfinpyrazone facilitate its excretion. Many doctors also prescribe anti-inflammatory colchicine, because gout medications may initially result in a worsening of symptoms.

Are gout medications available by prescription or over the counter?

Gout medications are available by prescription from your doctor.

What are the possible side effects of gout medications?

These vary from medication to medication. A common reaction to allopurinol is an initial increase in attacks of joint pain and swelling. Some other common side effects arc:

- Diarrhea

- Nausea

- Vomiting

- Stomach pain

- Hives

- Itching

- Liver function abnormalities

- Skin rash

- Sores

- Headache

- Loss of appetite

- Lowered blood count

Is there anyone who should *not* take gout medications?

Yes. Among the more common reasons to avoid these drugs are a history of kidney or liver disease, alcoholism, a low white blood cell or platelet count, or blood disease. Gout medications interact with many other drugs, so be sure to inform your doctor of all other drugs you are taking, whether prescription or over the counter.

OSTEOPOROSIS MEDICATIONS

Do traditional anti-inflammatory medications have an impact on osteoporosis?

If you break a vertebra or hip due to osteoporosis, your doctor may prescribe an NSAID. Otherwise NSAIDs have little or nothing to do with the disease process of osteoporosis.

Are there special medications for osteoporosis?

Yes. Medications to reduce bone loss form the basis of both the prevention and treatment of osteoporosis. Calcium and vitamin D supplements are also recommended if you don't take in enough of these nutrients in your regular diet.

Are people with arthritis at a special risk of developing osteoporosis?

Yes. If you take corticosteroid medications for rheumatoid arthritis, the resultant loss of bone mass can contribute to osteoporosis.

What are some examples of osteoporosis medications?

Following is a list of the major drugs for the treatment of osteoporosis. Medications are identified by their generic names followed by their brand names:

- Alendronate (Fosamax)

- Calcitonin injection (Calcimar, Miacalcin)

- Calcitonin nasal spray (Miacalcin)

- Conjugated estrogens (Premarin, Premphase, Prempro)

Are these all prescription medications?

Yes. These are powerful medications with many side effects, and although helpful in many cases they are not right for everyone. If you are a woman approaching menopause, or are otherwise at risk for osteoporosis, carefully explore all your treatment options with your physician.

TOPICAL MEDICATIONS

What are topical medications?

Unlike medications that are taken internally, creams, lotions, salves, sprays, and rubs are applied directly on sore areas of the body. They provide temporary relief of pain.

How do topical medications work?

They work in a number of different ways:

- By inhibiting prostaglandin production

- By stimulating or irritating local nerve endings, which distracts your brain from more major arthritis discomfort

- By depleting substances in the nerves that send pain messages to the brain

Who should use topical medications?

Topical medications are a good choice for people:

- Who suffer from muscle aches or mild pain that affects only a limited number of joints

- Whose other medications fail to completely manage pain

- Who cannot use other medications

Are there any special advantages to topical medications?

Since they are applied locally, topical medications reduce the incidence of systemic side effects.

What are the most common types of topical medications?

Topical medications most commonly contain combinations of the following:

- **Salicylates.** Salicylates inhibit the prostaglandins that lead to pain and inflammation. In addition, they decrease the ability of nerve endings in the skin to feel pain. Examples are Aspercreme and BenGay.

- **Counterirritants.** By stimulating or irritating local nerve endings, counterirritants distract the brain from the more major pain of arthritis. Examples include camphor, eucalyptus, oil of wintergreen, menthol, and turpentine.

- **Capsaicin.** A natural ingredient extracted from cayenne peppers, capsaicin works by depleting your body's supply of substance P, a neurotransmitter that passes pain messages to the brain. Examples include Zostrix and Zostrix HP.

THE COST OF MEDICATIONS

How much do arthritis medications cost?

Cost depends on a number of factors, including your dosage, the area of the country you live in, and the pharmacy you use. In addition, some health plans cover prescriptions and others don't. Generally speaking, generic versions of drugs—drugs that have been on the market for a long time—are less expensive than brand-name drugs.

My health care plan doesn't cover prescription drugs. Is there any other way of cutting my costs?

When cost is an issue, by all means be frank and open about this with your doctor. He or she may be able to help by giving you free samples left by drug company representatives. Alternatively, most drug companies provide a limited amount of medications for people who cannot otherwise afford them. Your doctor can tell you how to take advantage of these programs.

What about generic drugs?

Using generic drugs is another way to cut costs. Since whether a drug is available generically depends on how long it has been on the market, there are not yet generic versions of new COX-2 inhibitors.

SAFETY TIPS

- Take your medication exactly as prescribed or recommended by your doctor.

- Don't stop taking medication without first consulting your doctor.

- To avoid potentially dangerous interactions, always tell your doctor about all medications (both prescription and over the counter) that you are taking.

- Inform your doctor if you drink alcohol or take any illicit drugs.

- Let your doctor know if you are pregnant or breastfeeding.

- Tell your doctor at once if you experience any adverse reactions to a medication.

- Inform your doctor of any other medical conditions from which you are suffering, such as kidney or liver disease.

- Keep in mind that some drugs take longer to work than others.

TEN QUESTIONS YOU SHOULD ASK YOUR DOCTOR

Ask your doctor about any special instructions for taking your medication, such as:

1. What is the correct dose?

2. How and when should I take my medication?

3. What should I do if I miss a dose?

4. What are the benefits of this drug?

5. How quickly will it work?

6. What side effects should I expect?

7. Are there other drugs I should avoid while taking this medication?

8. When should I call the doctor if I don't experience relief?

9. If medication irritates my stomach, should I take it with food?

10. If I still experience gastrointestinal problems, what else can I do? Could COX-2 inhibitors be a better alternative?

PART II

The COX-2 Inhibitor Solution

FOUR

❖❖❖❖

The History of COX-2 Inhibitors

I'm not a medicine taker. In fact, I hate taking pills. But I'm in my second year of taking Celebrex and I'm 100 percent happy with it.

Laurie Stollery, 60-year-old osteoarthritis patient
and participant in Celebrex clinical trials

COX-2 inhibitors like Celebrex and Vioxx were designed by scientists to fill a need. It was clear for many years that, as valuable a role as they played in controlling arthritis pain and inflammation, ordinary nonselective NSAIDs had serious problems. For a time it was believed that nothing could be done about this. But about 10 years ago, researchers such as Dr. Philip Needleman began to suspect that there was a way of isolating the beneficial actions of NSAIDs from their unfortunate side effects on the gastrointestinal system. This was the beginning of the search for COX-2 inhibitors.

HOW COX-2 INHIBITORS CAME TO BE

What is the history of COX-2 inhibitors?

Dr. Philip Needleman, the Brooklyn-born scientist most responsible for bringing us Celebrex, the first FDA-approved COX-2 inhibitor, credits his discovery to a rabbit. Years ago at Washington University in St. Louis, he noticed that an inflamed rabbit kidney was furiously pumping out prostaglandins. This led him to hypothesize that inflamed cells produce a special type of prostaglandin, and Dr. Needleman became increasingly certain that this was because there were not one but two COX enzymes.

How were COX-2 inhibitors designed?

Scientists used advanced molecular technology to design COX-2 inhibitors like Celebrex. Once researchers like Dr. Needleman discovered that there were not one but two COX enzymes, the goal was to create a drug that blocked only the one involved in pain and inflammation. COX-2 inhibitors such as Celebrex and Vioxx were that drug.

How do COX-2 inhibitors work?

These drugs work by blocking or inhibiting only the COX 2 enzyme, the enzyme that triggers pain and inflammation. Therapeutic doses do not inhibit the COX 1 enzyme, which is left free to protect the stomach lining.

How is this action different from that of nonselective NSAIDs?

This is in contrast to NSAIDs in general, which inhibit both COX enzymes. Nonselective NSAIDs treat pain and inflammation but also are more likely than COX-2 inhibitors to damage the stomach lining. This can lead to ulcers, bleeding, and perforation.

What company makes Celebrex?

Celebrex is manufactured by G.D. Searle & Co., the pharmaceutical business unit of Monsanto at which Dr. Philip Needleman has been the chief scientist since 1991. It is being marketed jointly by Searle and Pfizer, the same company which launched pharmaceutical best-sellers Viagra and Lipitor.

Is there a great demand for COX-2 inhibitors?

Celebrex is the fastest-selling drug in U.S. history. In its first eight weeks on the market, nearly 900,000 prescriptions for Celebrex were written. In its first six months on the market, there were over seven million prescriptions. Celebrex sales have surpassed those of Pfizer's anti-impotence medication Viagra and the anti-cholesterol drug Lipitor, the previous best-sellers.

How frequently are COX-2 inhibitors prescribed for arthritis today?

COX-2 inhibitors already account for approximately one out of four prescriptions written for arthritis, second only to ibuprofen.

THE CLINICAL TRIALS

How do we know that COX-2 inhibitors are safe and effective?

Celebrex was tested in more than 13,000 people worldwide. In one of the most extensive arthritis clinical trial programs to date, volunteers enrolled in more than 50 different clinical studies in 23 countries.

That sounds like a lot of people to be involved in the testing of one drug. Is it?

Yes. Searle took the precaution of testing Celebrex in about 10 times the usual number of people involved in clinical trials.

How long have people been taking Celebrex in clinical trials?

Almost 2,500 people have been taking daily doses of between 200 and 800 milligrams for over a year.

How old were the people involved in the studies?

People ranged in age from 18 to 93.

What were some of the specific clinical trials used to test Celebrex?

- Three 12-week studies (two of the knee and one of the hip) in about 3,300 osteoarthritis (OA) patients compared different dosages of Celebrex with the highest commonly recommended dose of the prescription-strength NSAID naproxen and with a placebo.

- Two 6-week studies in some 1,400 OA patients contrasted a once-a-day dose of 200 milligrams of Celebrex to treatment with a placebo.

- Two 12-week studies of 2,250 rheumatoid arthritis (RA) patients compared different dosages of Celebrex with naproxen and with a placebo.

What were the results of these clinical trials?

Celebrex was demonstrated to be as effective as the highest commonly recommended dose of naproxen. In people who have osteoarthritis, Celebrex improved pain, stiffness, and activities such as walking, bending, and getting in and out of a car. And most important, while treating arthritis pain and inflammation just as effectively, Celebrex caused significantly fewer upper gastrointestinal ulcers than either naproxen and ibuprofen.

Did anyone in the Celebrex clinical trials experience minor gastrointestinal problems?

A small number of people experienced common GI side effects such as dyspepsia (stomach upset), diarrhea, and abdominal pain. But fewer than 1% left the trials as a result of these discomforts. Clinical trial participant Laurie Stollery of Rochester, New York, noted that there were a few people who chose to go off the study because of side effects, but then quickly wanted to come back on! Although this was against the rules of the clinical trial, they can now obtain Celebrex from their own physicians.

Did anyone in the clinical trials experience more serious GI problems?

In controlled clinical trials of mostly three months' duration, patients were given a daily dose of 200 or more milligrams of Celebrex. Two people out of 5,285 (or 0.04%) experienced significant upper GI bleeding at 14 and 22 days of beginning treatment.

Would that result be typical of Celebrex use?

Since about 40% of these people had medical tests which showed them to be free of ulcers at the beginning of this study, it's not clear how representative this sample is of the general population. More long-term studies are necessary to compare how often serious GI side effects take place in people who take Celebrex versus people who take other NSAIDs. Searle is continuing to conduct more wide-ranging COX-2 trials to find the answers to these questions.

THE CLINICAL TRIAL PARTICIPANTS

What were the experiences of some of the people who took Celebrex in the clinical trials?

Meet some of the participants:

- Thirty-seven-year-old Laurie Schuster of Illinois has suffered from osteoarthritis since her mid-twenties. Before she started taking Celebrex, stiffness forced Laurie to slowly and painfully roll herself out of bed each morning. Stairs were difficult if not impossible to negotiate. Arthritis affected Laurie professionally: She started working at temporary jobs because she could never be certain when her health would allow her to work. It affected her family life: Laurie couldn't visit family members who lived out of state, for sitting on a train or plane meant that her knees would be in agony during the trip and ache for days afterward. Day-to-day activities as well were difficult, the mechanics of shopping and cooking frustrating and sometimes not worth the trouble.

  Regular NSAIDs brought some relief to Laurie, but they irritated her stomach and sometimes she couldn't keep them down. After two weeks of taking Celebrex, however, Laurie was able to walk without the usual burning in the front of her calves. She feels "a thousand times better" today. What is only a twinge now would have meant walking with a cane in the not-so-distant past.

- Fifty-three-year-old Shirley Johnson is an entertainer in the Chicago area. Five or six years ago she developed osteoarthritis in her left knee. "It hindered me in a way," says Shirley, "since I couldn't do a lot of moving around on stage." In her second year of taking Celebrex, Shirley can now move to the music with no pain. Before seeing an ad for the Celebrex clinical trials on TV, she had been taking up to eight NSAIDs a day. "That eased the pain, but it didn't stop," she reports. "Celebrex took the pain away."

- Sixty-nine-year-old New Jersey resident Anne McFadden Pollack has had osteoarthritis for a little over 20 years. She also suffers from rheumatoid arthritis, although that is fortunately in remission. Anne's husband, Dave, a retired pharmacist, was a little nervous at first about her participating in clinical trials for a new drug. But Anne has been successfully taking Celebrex for the past year and a half with no side effects at all.

  "I still hurt," explains Anne, "but this takes more pain away. And the great thing is it doesn't hurt my stomach." Anne knows what she's talking about, for over the years she took a battery of NSAIDs for her arthritis, including Feldene, naproxen, and Daypro. Even though she took these NSAIDs with meals and special stomach-protective medications, she nonetheless developed an ulcer. Zantac helped, and fortunately Anne's ulcer had disappeared by the time she joined the Celebrex trials.

- After 36 years in the warehouse business, a debilitating combination of rheumatoid arthritis and osteoarthritis forced 57-year-old Frank Edwards of St. Louis into an early retirement. "I kind of gave up doing a lot of things," says Frank. "I didn't exercise because I hurt too bad. I couldn't reach things down on the floor because my knees were so swollen, and my fingers were so swollen I couldn't use the keyboard on the computer."

Stomach problems plagued Frank as he took NSAID after NSAID. "I had to watch what I ate," he explains. "If I took my medication on an empty stomach, I would throw up. Even if I ate breakfast first, the pills would still make me feel nauseous." For relief, Frank relied on everything from Tums and Alka-Seltzer to Pepcid and Zantac.

Things changed dramatically when Frank joined the clinical trials for Celebrex more than a year ago. After just a few days, he walked up the steps to his church instead of taking the elevator he had relied on for the preceding five years. And then, amazingly, Frank went back to work full time as the manager and buyer for another warehouse.

"I feel like I'm a new person since I started taking Celebrex," raves Frank. "I feel like I'm about 30 years old. Just recently I played basketball with my son for the first time in years. He said 'Whoa, Dad! You're back!' "

- Sixty-year-old Laurie Stollery of Rochester, New York, was diagnosed with osteoarthritis about four years ago. At first she wasn't sure what was wrong. But when a flare-up sent her to the emergency room, Laurie's regular doctor brought in a rheumatologist who made the diagnosis.

  Before getting involved in the Celebrex trials, Laurie took NSAIDs with Pepcid and Zantac to ease stomach problems. Now she no longer needs them. She's in her second year with Celebrex, and is 100% happy with it. Laurie also keeps active walking and bike riding, and feels that regular exercise helps keep her arthritis under control. She watches what she eats, keeps her weight down, and maintains a positive attitude. Most of all, Laurie tries to keep a lid on stress, the biggest trigger of her symptoms. "If something is bothering me for a week or two, I have to reprogram myself so I feel better," she says.

These stories are so encouraging. Is it possible that COX-2 inhibitors are a cure for arthritis?

No. There is no cure for arthritis. But COX-2 inhibitors can help you tame the pain and inflammation of this sometimes crippling disease. Most importantly, in therapeutic amounts they can accomplish this while causing fewer of the gastrointestinal side effects associated with nonsteroidal anti-inflammatory drugs ordinarily prescribed for the purpose.

But the stories of the clinical trial participants make it sound as though Celebrex controlled their pain and inflammation more effectively. Why is that?

In clinical trials, Celebrex and other NSAIDs met with equal success in controlling pain and inflammation. Again, the major advantage was that Celebrex significantly reduced the incidence of ulcers. But some arthritis sufferers undoubtedly experience more relief from some medications rather than others. That is true of the arthritis sufferers whose stories you read here.

Why do experts think this happens?

It's possible that quality of life issues play a role. "When you don't have stomach problems and you're not worried about getting them, you have a better quality of life," explains Dr. Peter C. Isakson, who leads COX-2 technology Research and Development at Searle. "This might make you feel better."

Patients' expectations too may play a role in how effective drugs appear to be. Dr. Isakson thinks that another part of the answer could be that their doctors told them they might feel better with the new medication, and so they did.

Dr. Jay Goldstein of the University of Illinois, who was closely involved in the clinical trials of Celebrex, speculates that perhaps because patients taking a COX-2 inhibitor don't experience upset stomachs or ulcers and moreover have no fear of developing them, they are more likely to stick to their medication schedule and thus experience greater pain relief.

FIVE

◆◆◆◆

COX-2 Inhibitors:
The Stomach-Friendly Alternative

Celebrex is the best thing that ever happened to me. When I was taking other medications, I used to have to watch everything ate. Now I can eat barbecued food or sauerkraut or anything else I want. I'm pain-free, I'm heartburn-free, and I have no side effects whatsoever. I feel like a whole new person.

Frank Edwards, 57-year-old osteoarthritis and rheumatoid arthritis patient and participant in Celebrex clinical trials

Like many people who do battle with chronic disease, you may be filled with questions and doubts about medications. Even if you suffer from uncomfortable and potentially even life-threatening side effects such as bleeding ulcers, you may feel hesitant about switching to a new and unfamiliar remedy. Is it safe? How is it different from other arthritis drugs? How do you know if it's right for you? In this chapter, you will learn the answers to these and many other questions about COX-2 inhibitors.

HOW COX-2 INHIBITORS ARE DIFFERENT

Why is everyone so excited about these new drugs?

There are millions of arthritis sufferers, both in this country and abroad. Some are happy with their treatment, but many others are frustrated in their efforts to control pain and inflammation without suffering adverse side effects. And so it comes as no surprise that COX-2 inhibitors—as effective as standard nonsteroidal anti-inflammatory painkillers but with fewer of their stomach-damaging side effects—have attracted worldwide attention. Experts speculate that the arrival of COX-2 inhibitors may usher in a whole new era in arthritis treatment.

How do we know that COX-2 inhibitors are safe medications?

COX-2 inhibitors have undergone extensive research, investigation, and clinical trials. For example, it was only after careful consideration and lengthy meetings with its manufacturer, G.D. Searle, that the Food and Drug Administration (FDA) approved Celebrex for the treatment of osteoarthritis and rheumatoid arthritis.

When were COX-2 inhibitors approved by the FDA?

Celebrex, placed on a special fast track for consideration by the FDA, was approved on December 30, 1998. Vioxx received final approval from the FDA on May 21, 1999. In its first six months on the market, Celebrex eclipsed Viagra to become the fastest-selling new drug ever.

What kinds of arthritis are COX-2 inhibitors prescribed for?

The FDA approved Celebrex for relief of the signs and symptoms of osteoarthritis (OA) and adult rheumatoid arthritis (RA). Vioxx has been approved for OA and acute general and menstrual pain.

How is Celebrex helpful in the treatment of arthritis?

All research indicates that Celebrex significantly reduces joint pain and stiffness in arthritis patients without, in the vast majority of cases, causing gastrointestinal side effects. In clinical trials, Celebrex improved patients' abilities to perform everyday functions such as walking, bending, and getting in and out of cars.

What is it that makes COX-2 inhibitors like Celebrex and Vioxx different from other arthritis medications?

Because COX-2 inhibitors are more *selective* in their actions than ordinary nonsteroidal anti-inflammatory medications (NSAIDs), in most cases therapeutic doses can make you feel better without upsetting your stomach or causing dangerous ulcers.

Does this mean that COX-2 inhibitors are safer than other NSAIDs?

We don't know the answer to this question yet, for only time will tell. We do know that Celebrex is different from other NSAIDs based on its lack of platelet effects and a lower incidence of GI ulcers. Whether that translates into a true "safety" benefit has yet to be proven.

Are COX-2 inhibitors as effective as other arthritis medications in controlling pain and inflammation?

Yes. In clinical trials the effectiveness of Celebrex and Vioxx was comparable to that of NSAIDs such as naproxen and ibuprofen.

Does Celebrex go by any other names?

The generic name for Celebrex is celecoxib.

What is Celebrex made of?

Celebrex (celecoxib) is chemically designated as 4-[5-(4-methylphenyl)-3-(trifluoromethyl)-1H-pyrazol-1-yl] benzenesulfonamide and is a diaryl substituted pyrazole. The empirical formula for celecoxib is $C_{17}H_{14}F_3N_3O_2S$, and the molecular weight is 381.38. Celebrex oral capsules contain 100 mg and 200 mg of celecoxib. The inactive ingredients in Celebrex capsules include: croscarmellose sodium, edible inks, gelatin, lactose monohydrate, magnesium stearate, povidone, sodium lauryl sulfate, and titanium dioxide.

How can I get COX-2 inhibitors?

Celebrex and Vioxx are available by prescription only. If other NSAIDs are causing stomach problems for you, ask your doctor about COX-2 inhibitors.

Do COX-2 inhibitors have any other uses beyond treatment of OA and RA?

Vioxx has been approved for acute general and menstrual pain. COX-2 inhibitors such as Celebrex and Vioxx may eventually be approved by the FDA for a wider range of uses. In the meantime, they may be prescribed on an off-label basis for other health problems.

What does "off-label" mean?

In order to receive timely approval from the FDA, a pharmaceutical company ordinarily applies for the approval of a drug to treat a distinct medical problem. Once the FDA has approved that drug as safe, doctors are free to prescribe it on an "off-label basis" to treat other conditions, despite the fact that the drug does not have specific FDA approval for those ailments.

HOW COX-2 INHIBITORS WORK

How do COX-2 inhibitors like Celebrex and Vioxx work?

COX-2 inhibitors ease the pain and swelling of arthritis by blocking an enzyme in the body called COX 2. COX stands for cyclooxygenase, an enzyme that helps make prostaglandins, the substances that are largely responsible for the joint pain and inflammation of arthritis. Prostaglandins make nerve endings more sensitive and thus intensify pain.

How are COX-2 inhibitors different from nonselective NSAIDs?

New COX-2 inhibitors like Celebrex and Vioxx are specially designed to prevent the gastrointestinal disturbances associated with nonselective NSAIDs. Like them, COX-2 inhibitors exert an anti-inflammatory effect by blocking the COX 2 enzyme. But there are two COX enzymes in our bodies—COX 1 and COX 2—and COX-2 inhibitors are more selective in their actions on these enzymes than ordinary NSAIDs. When used at therapeutic doses, Celebrex and Vioxx block only the COX 2 enzyme that leads to pain and inflammation. Less selective NSAIDs such as prescription Daypro and Naprosyn or over-the-counter Advil and Motrin also deplete the COX-1 enzyme that protects the stomach lining, and as a result are more frequently associated with serious side effects such as ulcers and gastrointestinal bleeding.

Does this mean that the COX 1 and COX 2 enzymes have different functions?

Yes, typically they do.

What is the function of the COX 1 enzyme?

COX 1 protects your stomach lining. Blocking it—as aspirin, ibuprofen, and other conventional NSAIDs do—can lead to GI problems such as bleeding and ulcers.

Does the COX 1 enzyme have any other functions?

Yes. COX 1 is also closely involved in platelet function. Platelets are substances in the blood that are involved in a process called hemostasis. This means that they become sticky—or in medical terms, they "aggregate"—when you cut yourself. They form a blood clot, like a small patch, to protect the injured area.

What is the function of the COX 2 enzyme?

COX 2 is the enzyme responsible for the pain and inflammation of arthritis.

COX-2 INHIBITORS AND OTHER NSAIDS

Are COX-2 inhibitors such as Celebrex and Vioxx NSAIDs?

COX-2 inhibitors including Celebrex and Vioxx are a subcategory of NSAIDs. Like NSAIDs, the most commonly used medications for arthritis, COX-2 inhibitors help control the pain and inflammation of arthritis. Unfortunately, conventional NSAIDs appear more likely to cause uncomfortable and sometimes even dangerous gastrointestinal side effects. Because their actions in your body are more selective, COX-2 inhibitors such as Celebrex and Vioxx are associated with fewer side effects than ordinary NSAIDs.

What exactly is a COX-2 inhibitor?

A COX-2 inhibitor is a new type of NSAID that works by selectively blocking or inhibiting the enzyme known as COX 2. COX 2 plays an important role in the pain and inflammation of arthritis. By blocking COX 2, you block pain and inflammation.

Importantly, however, COX-2 inhibitors block only COX 2. They do not block the COX 1 enzyme, which because of its protective effects on the stomach and other positive actions in the body is nicknamed "the housekeeping enzyme." Because COX-2 inhibitors block only COX 2 and leave COX 1 alone, scientists refer to them as "COX-1 sparing."

I keep hearing that COX-2 inhibitors are "selective" NSAIDs. What does that mean?

In therapeutic doses, COX-2 inhibitors like Celebrex and Vioxx block or inhibit only the COX 2 enzyme involved in pain and inflammation. COX-2 inhibitors do not affect the housekeeping COX 1 enzyme, which goes on to perform its positive, protective actions in the body. This is in contrast to ordinary nonselective NSAIDs, which block both the COX 1 and the COX 2 enzymes, and therefore control pain and inflammation but can also lead to stomach problems. Because of their more selective actions in the body, Celebrex and Vioxx are known as selective COX-2 inhibitors.

What are the pros and cons of NSAIDs?

"NSAIDs are a double-edged sword," explains Dr. Jay Goldstein, a board-certified gastroenterologist and associate professor of medicine at the University of Illinois at Chicago. They give patients a better quality of life by reducing pain and inflammation, but cause gastrointestinal side effects including dyspepsia (upset stomach), ulcers, and complications of ulcers (most commonly, bleeding, obstruction, and perforation). Symptomatic ulcers—ulcers that cause pain—occur in 2% to 4% of those who take nonselective NSAIDs.

Did the clinical trials demonstrate that COX-2 inhibitors caused fewer ulcers than nonselective NSAIDs?

Yes. In order to ensure that their results were as accurate as possible, doctors used a procedure called an endoscopy to peer into the stomachs of trial participants. Endoscopies revealed fewer ulcers in patients treated with Celebrex.

How serious are the problems with ordinary NSAIDs?

The problems are serious, and sometimes even fatal:

- Of the 13 million people who use NSAIDs such as ibuprofen each year, up to 5% have severe stomach problems. Fifteen percent experience milder side effects such as heartburn or nausea.

- About 107,000 people are hospitalized each year for upper gastrointestinal or GI complications of NSAID use.

- Every year, 16,500 patients die from GI complications due to NSAID use.

- Annual costs for hospitalizations from serious side effects of NSAID use are over $1 billion.

Can COX-2 inhibitors control arthritis pain and inflammation any more effectively than nonselective NSAIDs?

No. COX-2 inhibitors such as Celebrex and Vioxx control pain and inflammation *as* effectively, but not more effectively, than nonselective NSAIDs. The major difference between nonselective NSAIDs and selective COX-2 inhibitors is that COX-2 inhibitors cause fewer gastrointestinal side effects.

I've heard Celebrex called "the new super aspirin." Is that a good nickname for this medication?

For a variety of reasons, no. Celebrex is *not* aspirin. Aspirin and Celebrex are similar in that both relieve pain and inflammation. But they also have very different properties:

• Unlike aspirin, therapeutic doses of Celebrex are not likely to cause gastrointestinal problems such as ulcers. While aspirin is the prototype NSAID, RA patients must take relatively high doses (8 or more a day).

• It would be unfortunate and misleading for people to take Celebrex thinking that it has the same heart-protective effect as aspirin. It doesn't.

If heart disease runs in my family or I'm otherwise at risk of cardiovascular problems, should I take aspirin instead of COX-2 inhibitors like Celebrex or Vioxx?

Only your own physician can answer that question for sure, but the answer will probably be that you can take both. You may be instructed to take a COX-2 inhibitor for your arthritis, and a baby aspirin a day for cardiovascular protection.

THE POTENTIAL SIDE EFFECTS

I've heard that COX-2 inhibitors don't cause side effects. Is this true?

No. No drug, however safe, is completely free of side effects.

What types of side effects do COX-2 inhibitors cause?

Because COX-2 inhibitors block only the COX-2 enzyme, at therapeutic doses they cause only minimal side effects. While they cannot completely eliminate your risk of possible side effects such as diarrhea, stomach bleeding, and ulcers, COX-2 inhibitors can reduce them.

To what extent do COX-2 inhibitors reduce my risk of gastrointestinal side effects?

Clinical studies demonstrated a fourfold decrease in ulcers in patients who used Celebrex, in comparison to those who used nonselective NSAIDs.

Should people who take COX-2 inhibitors be on the lookout for possible gastrointestinal problems?

Absolutely. Although COX-2 inhibitors have a lower potential for stomach problems, these side effects can occur. As with other NSAIDs, serious GI problems such as bleeding and ulcers are insidious and can creep up on you without warning.

What can I do to avoid GI problems?

To minimize your risk, the lowest effective dose should be taken for the shortest possible time.

Are there any other precautions I can take to avoid GI problems?

As with conventional NSAIDs, there are some helpful steps you can take:

• Alert your doctor promptly if you experience any gastrointestinal problems.

• To be on the safe side, have regular checkups. Be

aware that ulcers and internal bleeding can occur without your even knowing about it.

Are there any other common side effects?

Outside of gastrointestinal problems, the most commonly reported side effects were headache, upper respiratory infection, and sinusitis.

WHEN CAUTION SHOULD BE EXERCISED

Is there anyone who should avoid taking COX-2 inhibitors?

Yes. Do not take Celebrex:

- If you have a known hypersensitivity to celecoxib

- If you have experienced an allergic reaction to sulfonamides

- If you are allergic to aspirin or other NSAIDs

I have a history of diarrhea and stomach pain. Does this put me at a higher risk of developing GI problems while taking COX-2 inhibitors?

Yes. All NSAIDs, including Celebrex and Vioxx, should be used with caution in those who have a prior history of ulcer disease or gastrointestinal bleeding.

Studies show that these people have a greater than tenfold higher risk of developing a GI bleed.

Are there any other conditions that increase my risk of GI bleeding?

In addition to a prior history of ulcer disease, other conditions that may increase your risk of gastrointestinal bleeding are:

• Treatment with oral corticosteroids

• Treatment with anticoagulants

• Longer duration of NSAID therapy

• Smoking

• Alcoholism

• Older age

• Poor general health status

Who is at the highest risk of death from gastrointestinal complications?

The elderly and debilitated are at the greatest risk. Because of this, NSAIDs of all kinds should only be used with extreme caution in these people.

Is there any danger of anaphylaxis due to COX-2 inhibitors such as Celebrex?

Anaphylaxis is a rare allergic reaction to NSAIDs that involves difficulty in breathing and swallowing, dizziness, fainting, hives, a fast or irregular heartbeat, or a swollen tongue and puffy eyelids. There is no greater risk of anaphylaxis with COX-2 inhibitors than with any other NSAIDs, and there were no instances of anaphylaxis in the Celebrex clinical trials. To be on the safe side, however, COX-2 inhibitors should not be taken if you have asthma along with rhinitis (with or without nasal polyps) or have experienced severe bronchospasm after taking aspirin or other NSAIDs. If anaphylaxis is ever suspected, emergency help should be sought at once.

I have kidney disease as well as arthritis. Is it safe for me to take COX-2 inhibitors?

Since clinical trials are routinely conducted with otherwise healthy participants, no information is available about the use of COX-2 inhibitors in those who have advanced renal disease. Therefore, treatment with COX-2 inhibitors is not recommended. If it is undertaken, kidney function should be very closely monitored.

Do COX-2 inhibitors have any effect on fertility?

In animal studies, Celebrex had no effect on fertility.

Can COX-2 inhibitors be safely taken during pregnancy? Will they harm my unborn child?

It's best not to take any medication whatsoever when you are pregnant, for every food you eat and drug you take is passed on to your developing fetus through the placenta. While COX-2 inhibitors have obviously not been tested in pregnant women, research in animals indicates that they should in particular be avoided in late pregnancy.

Is it safe to take COX-2 inhibitors while breastfeeding?

As during pregnancy, it's best to avoid all medications when breastfeeding. In this case, substances you ingest are passed on to your growing baby via your breast milk. If your arthritis symptoms are so severe and disabling that medication is required, you should discuss with your doctor whether it is safe to continue breastfeeding or whether you should switch your baby to formula.

Can children take COX-2 inhibitors?

Not at this point. For instance, Celebrex use has not yet been investigated in anyone under the age of 18. Clinical trials always focus first on adults, since we always want to be most protective of our children.

Will children be able to take COX-2 inhibitors at some point in the future?

It's possible. Searle, the company that makes Celebrex, is working with the FDA on making this drug available to children who suffer from juvenile RA.

DRUG INTERACTIONS

What drug interactions should I be aware of when taking COX-2 inhibitors such as Celebrex or Vioxx?

COX-2 inhibitors interact with a number of other drugs, including the following:

- **Ace-inhibitors.** NSAIDs may diminish the antihypertensive effects of ACE inhibitors (angiotensin converting enzyme inhibitors).

- **Furosemide.** NSAIDs can reduce the effect of furosemide and thiazides.

- **Aspirin.** Celebrex can be used with low dose aspirin. However, using aspirin along with Celebrex may result in an increased risk of gastrointestinal ulcerations or other complications, compared to the use of Celebrex alone. Because they do not have the same effect on platelets, COX-2 inhibitors are not a substitute for aspirin as far as its heart-protective effects are concerned.

- **Fluconazole.** Because fluconazole increases the amount of Celebrex in the blood, those who take fluconazole should take the lowest possible dose of Celebrex.

- **Lithium.** Celebrex increases the level of lithium in the blood. People who are taking lithium should be carefully monitored if they also take COX-2 inhibitors.

- **Warfarin.** Caution should be exercised when taking COX-2 inhibitors along with warfarin, because people taking warfarin are at an increased risk of bleeding complications.

COST CONSIDERATIONS

How much do COX-2 inhibitors cost? Is their cost comparable to that of other arthritis medications?

Celebrex costs users about $2.50 a day, or about $75 for a one-month prescription. By contrast, generic ibuprofen costs about $24. However, the higher cost of COX-2 inhibitors doesn't appear to be discouraging arthritis sufferers who want pain relief with fewer side effects.

Will my insurance plan cover the cost of COX-2 inhibitors?

This depends on your health plan. However, if your doctor demonstrates that you have experienced stomach problems while taking other NSAIDs, your health plan should cover the cost of COX-2 inhibitors like Celebrex and Vioxx.

HOW TO TAKE COX-2 INHIBITORS

What is the recommended therapeutic dose of COX-2 inhibitors?

If you have OA, the recommended therapeutic dose of Celebrex is 200 milligrams daily, taken as a single dose, or 100 milligrams twice a day. For RA, the recommended Celebrex dose is 100 to 200 milligrams twice daily. Most people find it more convenient to take medication just once a day, when this is possible. (Vioxx, approved for the treatment of OA but not RA, is taken just once a day.)

If I still experience discomfort, should I take a higher doses of COX-2 inhibitors?

No. You should always take COX-2 inhibitors, and for that matter any drug, precisely as prescribed by your doctor.

I've been taking COX-2 inhibitors for some time, and my pain and swelling are under control. Does this mean that I can stop taking my medication?

Absolutely not. The most probable reason that your arthritis is under control is precisely because you are regularly taking your medication. To stop would most likely mean a return of symptoms.

Does it matter whether I take COX-2 inhibitors once or twice a day?

If you have rheumatoid arthritis, Celebrex should be taken twice a day. If you have osteoarthritis, ask your physician if it is possible for you to take only one dose daily. Vioxx is taken once daily for OA.

How long does it take for COX-2 inhibitors to take effect?

The OA trials showed that pain relief was apparent one to two days after beginning to take Celebrex, and was maximum after seven days.

Should I take COX-2 inhibitors with meals? Does this make any difference?

Since COX-2 inhibitors are less likely than other NSAIDs to lead to stomach upset, it is less important to take it with meals. However, to be on the safe side, it's still a good idea to take COX-2 inhibitors with food.

Will taking Celebrex for long periods cause any long-term damage?

Not that we know of. But keep in mind that COX-2 inhibitors have only recently been approved by the FDA. While they seem relatively safe, only time will tell for certain.

Is it possible to take an overdose of COX-2 inhibitors?

Although this did not occur in clinical trials, it is possible (although not likely) to overdose on any NSAID. The symptoms of overdose are lethargy, drowsiness, nausea, and painful vomiting. GI bleeding can also occur. In rare cases, there may be hypertension, acute renal failure, respiratory depression, and coma. If you suspect an overdose, go immediately to the nearest emergency room.

POTENTIAL FUTURE USES

What is the future for COX-2 inhibitors like Celebrex and Vioxx?

COX-2 inhibitors have been specifically approved for relief of the signs and symptoms of osteoarthritis (Celebrex and Vioxx) and adult rheumatoid arthritis

(Celebrex alone). Vioxx has also been approved for acute general and menstrual pain. In time scientists expect it to be applied to a far wider range of uses.

What role may COX-2 inhibitors play as an analgesia or pain reliever?

Vioxx (although not Celebrex) has been approved by the FDA for acute general and menstrual pain.

Can COX-2 inhibitors ease dental pain?

In clinical trials COX-2 inhibitors relieved dental pain, which is medically viewed as an especially tough and persistent type of pain to control. Vioxx can be used to treat acute general pain.

What about postsurgical pain?

Again, Vioxx can be used to relieve acute general pain.

Can COX-2 inhibitors play a role in the treatment of menstrual pain?

Vioxx has been approved for the treatment of menstrual pain. "I used to sneak an occasional Celebrex for menstrual pain and it worked great," reports Laurie Schuster, 37-year-old osteoarthritis patient and participant in Celebrex clinical trials.

What about backaches? Can COX-2 inhibitors ease this type of pain?

Vioxx has been approved by the FDA for the relief of acute general pain such as backaches.

I've heard that someday COX-2 inhibitors may be helpful in the treatment of Alzheimer's disease. Is this true?

The evidence at this point is strictly unofficial, but research does suggest that COX-2 inhibitors may slow the progression of this devastating disease. The level of COX-2 activity is heightened in those who suffer from Alzheimer's disease, so it is logical that taking a COX-2 inhibitor can block the activity of this enzyme and thus have a preventive effect.

Are there any studies that show this?

In an epidemiological study at Johns Hopkins, people who took ibuprofen had a significantly reduced chance of developing Alzheimer's disease. Since COX-2 inhibitors can block COX 2 with a lower incidence of GI side effects, the thinking is that they can accomplish the same objective in a safer manner. Searle, the company that makes Celebrex, currently has one trial underway with results expected at the end of 1999, but at least one more trial will be needed to demonstrate the effectiveness of COX-2 inhibitors in this disease.

Can COX-2 inhibitors help prevent colon cancer?

In the early 1990s, evidence first came to light suggesting that COX-2 inhibitors might play a role in preventing colon cancer. Epidemiology records in Tennessee showed that rheumatoid arthritis patients had a 40% to 50% lower chance of developing colon cancer. Since that time, more than 20 other studies have suggested that NSAIDs taken for the pain and inflammation of rheumatoid arthritis might offer a significant protective effect against colon cancer and polyps. (Polyps are often the precursors of colon cancer.)

Is there any further proof of this?

Animal studies have also indicated that COX-2 inhibitors may help prevent colon cancer, and Searle is conducting studies of its own to determine Celebrex's protective effects. "We'll be talking to the FDA very soon about the anticancer potential of Celebrex," confirms Dr. Peter C. Isakson, who leads COX-2 technology Research and Development at Searle.

Do COX-2 inhibitors have potential in the prevention of any other types of cancer?

Yes, they do. Extremely exciting research shows that there are other forms of cancer—notably skin cancer and bladder cancer—that involve COX 2.

Are COX-2 inhibitors likely to be prescribed on an off-label basis?

Pharmaceutical companies typically apply to the FDA for approval of a drug to treat one medical problem at a time. Yet once the FDA has approved or labeled that drug as safe for the original symptom or disease, it may be used to treat other conditions as well. Although the pharmaceutical company will in most likelihood apply for approval to treat these other conditions, it may be a number of years before this takes place. In the meantime, physicians can prescribe these drugs as they judge necessary on an off-label basis.

MORE COX-2 INHIBITORS ON THE HORIZON

In addition to Celebrex and Vioxx, are there any other COX-2 inhibitors in the works?

Yes. Since there is a $5 billion-a-year market for pain-killing drugs, not surprisingly a host of other pharmaceutical companies are racing to create and market their own versions of COX-2 inhibitors:

- Germany's Boehringer Ingelheim GmbH is set to launch its own COX-2 inhibitor, Mobic, later this year. Mobic will be co-marketed in this country with Abbott Laboratories.

- Glaxo Wellcome, a British company which is the second largest drug manufacturer in the world, also has a COX-2 inhibitor in the works.

Is this to the benefit of arthritis sufferers?

Yes. This is really excellent news for consumers, who will have an increasing number of treatment options to choose from.

Have any trials comparing the various COX-2 inhibitors taken place?

No head-to-head trials have been conducted as yet.

What were some of the specific clinical trials used to test Vioxx?

* In people who had osteoarthritis of the knee and hip, Vioxx improved physical functioning and reduced pain and inflammation. Vioxx was generally well tolerated in these trials, and no serious gastrointestinal side effects were reported.

* In a six-week pilot study, Vioxx reduced pain and inflammation in people with rheumatoid arthritis.

* In two separate dental pain studies, Vioxx relieved postsurgery dental pain as effectively as naproxen sodium and ibuprofen. These two NSAIDs are commonly used to relieve moderate to severe pain.

- In comparison to ibuprofen and a placebo, Vioxx gave greater relief of menstrual pain.

- Healthy volunteers who took a dose 10 times higher than normal experienced no more GI problems than those taking a placebo.

SIX
◆◆◆◆

Managing the Pain

My hands used to be so sore that I hated to have to shake hands with anyone. Now that I'm taking Celebrex, they still hurt but the pain is much less.

Anne McFadden Pollack, 69-year-old
osteoarthritis patient and participant in
Celebrex clinical trials

Pain can be your constant companion when you have arthritis. Even when you are not actually experiencing it, pain may interfere with the rhythm of your day-to-day life as you take precautions to ward off its next flare. Medication, a good balance of rest and exercise, a positive attitude, and a variety of self-help techniques can go far toward helping you get on top of pain. In cases of severe and persistent pain that fails to respond to other measures and seriously impairs your quality of life, surgery is a last resort.

Does pain have the same impact on everyone with arthritis?

No. First of all, it depends on what type of arthritis you have. Some people have intensely painful inflammatory arthritis that significantly interferes with day-to-day activities. Others have mild aches and pains for years without even realizing they have the disease. Then too each one of us experiences pain in our own unique fashion. Some of us are oblivious to all but the most intense pain, while others are sensitive to the tiniest twinge. The important thing to realize is that there are no rights and wrongs when it comes to pain. Pain is an individual experience.

What causes arthritis pain?

A number of factors are involved:

* Inflammation of the joint linings that leads to redness and swelling

* Tissue damage resulting from inflammation, injury, deterioration, or pressure on joints

* Muscle strain, as overworked muscles struggle to compensate for weakened joints

* Fatigue, a component of arthritis that can make pain seem even worse

Do psychological factors affect pain?

Absolutely. If you are sitting around the house thinking about how unlucky you are to have arthritis, the pain may feel virtually unbearable. If you are isolated from friends and family, you may find yourself dwelling on pain and experiencing it more intensely.

On the other hand, if like arthritis sufferer Laurie Stollery you have a positive attitude, you can control your pain instead of letting it control you. "I'm a positive thinking person," explains Laurie, who is retired from Eastman Kodak and lives in Rochester, New York. "I have arthritis and I do what I need to do to deal with it. I exercise, watch what I eat, and take Celebrex to control the pain. Then I just get on with my life." To that end, Laurie at age 60 still works part time, enjoys bicycling, and walks 6 miles a week.

Does this mean that pain is all in my head?

Not at all. Pain is a very real and sometimes very intrusive manifestation of arthritis. There may be occasions when all the positive thinking in the world is going to have zero impact on intense arthritis pain. That's why there are plenty of other options, including pain medications, range-of-motion exercises, heat and cold treatments, and even surgery.

What should I do if my doctor doesn't take my pain seriously?

This happened to Celebrex user Laurie Schuster, who developed osteoarthritis at a young age. "When

I was 25 years old, I was in constant pain," explains Laurie. "But no one took me seriously, and my doctor didn't want to give me painkillers." Now that she is taking Celebrex, Laurie's pain is under control. If your pain is not taken seriously, it's time to look for a new doctor.

I feel more pain when I'm anxious or depressed. Is this normal?

Yes. When you feel anxious or depressed, life can seem overwhelming and pain appears more intense.

In what way do emotions have an impact on pain?

When you suffer from a painful, chronic disease, emotional turmoil often accompanies your increasing physical challenges and limitations. You may feel unhappy about your declining abilities and yearn for the way things used to be. Friends and family may consciously or unconsciously feel the same way, and despite their good intentions place demands on you to perform actions of which you are no longer capable. Riding this emotional roller coaster, it's easy to become locked into an unhealthy pattern of dwelling too much on physical limitations, which leads to depression, which leads to more pain, which leads to stress, which leads to dwelling on physical limitations, and so on. Use the strategies you read about in this chapter to break this pattern.

My arthritis bothers me more when I'm run down. Is there any way around this?

Yes. Getting a good balance of exercise and rest is essential to everyone's overall health, but it's especially important when you suffer from a chronic disease. Fatigue is a physical component of arthritis, and you must take positive steps to deal with it. Listen to your body's signals. If your joints ache and you can't keep your eyes open, take a nap.

But what does fatigue have to do with arthritis?

Living with a chronic disease can be an emotionally exhausting experience. In addition, the systemic inflammation of certain kinds of arthritis (such as rheumatoid arthritis and lupus) and the poor sleep patterns typical of fibromyalgia are physical causes of fatigue.

How can I best manage fatigue?

The strategies you learn about in this chapter can help you simultaneously manage the pain, stress, and fatigue of arthritis. For example, getting a good night's sleep provides you with the energy to deal with pain and gives your joints a rest. Taking medication, learning to pace yourself, balancing exercise and rest, involving your family, and using your time and energy more efficiently are among the many steps you can take to overcome fatigue.

My cousin manages her arthritis pain with just aspirin and exercise, but this doesn't work for me. Should I be concerned?

Absolutely not. Every person is unique not only in how she experience pain but also in how she copes with it. What works for your cousin will not necessarily work for you, and vice versa. The important thing is to work with your health-care team to devise the pain management plan that works for you.

Does pain serve any real purpose in the body?

Yes. Pain is your body's way of warning you that something is wrong. When you touch something sharp or hot, your nerves rush chemical messengers carrying this information to the brain. In response to this acute pain, your brain fires a rapid message back to quickly withdraw your hand from danger.

What about the pain of arthritis?

In contrast to acute pain, the pain of arthritis is chronic. Arthritis pain can be severe and persistent, forcing you to endure it for long periods of time. This chronic pain is not as easily resolved as the acute variety, but in order to enjoy a good quality of life you must formulate a plan to cope with it.

How do our bodies physically block pain?

Your brain releases chemicals called endorphins to block pain signals. Many different actions can influence the production of these natural painkillers. Spending time with loved ones, engaging in a favorite hobby, and exercising are three simple things you can do to stimulate the release of morphine-like endorphins. Taking a walk on the beach or through the woods can also help. Medically speaking, medications such as codeine work by inducing the body to produce endorphins, as do self-care measures such as heat and cold treatments.

MEDICATIONS

What medications are used to control the pain of arthritis?

In many cases, over-the-counter medications such as Tylenol, Advil, Excedrin, or Aleve ease the pain of arthritis. If you find that these are sufficient to manage your pain, consider yourself fortunate. You have no need for stronger prescription drugs.

My arthritis continues to bother me no matter how many over-the-counter remedies I take. What should I do?

See your doctor. If your pain is persistent or severe, stronger pain medications are available by prescription.

What medications are most commonly prescribed to relieve arthritis pain?

Nonsteroidal anti-inflammatory drugs, or NSAIDs, are the main line of medicinal offense against pain.

Some NSAIDs are available over the counter, while others are available by prescription only. Common NSAIDs include aspirin, ibuprofen, naproxen sodium, oxaprozin, and piroxicam. (For further information, consult the list of NSAIDs in Chapter Three.)

What about codeine and other narcotics? Are they ever prescribed for arthritis?

Yes, but because of their addictive nature, drugs like codeine and morphine are prescribed with caution.

How safe and effective are NSAIDs?

NSAIDs, the most commonly used medications for arthritis, can relieve pain and inflammation, thus improving your overall quality of life. Unfortunately, NSAIDs can also have uncomfortable and sometimes even dangerous gastrointestinal side effects. Fifty-three-year-old entertainer Shirley Johnson entered the Celebrex clinical trials when she found that she was taking up to eight aspirins a day to relieve arthritis pain. This can be very hard on the stomach. While COX-2 inhibitors can't completely eliminate GI complications, they reduce their likelihood. In nearly two years of taking Celebrex, Shirley has experienced no stomach problems nor any other side effects.

What are the most common side effects of NSAIDs?

Stomach irritation and ulcers are most common.

Is there anything I can do to prevent stomach irritation when taking NSAIDs?

Fortunately, there is. Always take NSAIDs with meals, a glass of milk, or an antacid. Munching a few crackers or a slice of bread along with your medication is a helpful way to prevent stomach upset. Avoid alcohol when taking these medications, which can increase your risk of ulcers and stomach bleeding. If you do experience any gastrointestinal problems, see your doctor promptly.

Will everyone who takes NSAIDs experience uncomfortable side effects?

No. Although it's important to be aware of the possible side effects of any medication that you take, hopefully you will experience no side effects at all.

My stomach feels fine. Do I still have to worry about side effects?

Even though you feel fine, it's best to have regular checkups when taking NSAIDs. Ulcers and internal bleeding are deceptive conditions that can develop without your even knowing about them.

When are COX-2 inhibitors a better alternative for pain relief?

For those who experience gastrointestinal side effects such as ulcers, COX-2 inhibitors such as Celebrex and Vioxx may be a better alternative.

What exactly are COX-2 inhibitors?

These are new medications that are more selective than ordinary or nonselective NSAIDs in how they affect your body.

Are COX-2 inhibitors a special type of NSAID?

As of this time, the FDA has designated COX-2 inhibitors to be a subcategory of NSAIDs. COX-2 inhibitors are sometimes referred to as the selective NSAIDs.

Are COX-2 inhibitors very new drugs?

Yes. It was only on December 30, 1998 that the Food and Drug Administration (FDA) approved Celebrex, the first stomach-friendly COX-2 inhibitor to relieve the pain and inflammation of arthritis. Vioxx was approved on May 21, 1999.

How do we know that COX-2 inhibitors are safe?

Searle, the company that makes Celebrex, tested it in more than 13,000 people worldwide. This is about 10 times the usual number of people involved in clinical trial results submitted to the FDA. The studies showed that Celebrex relieved arthritis pain and inflammation as effectively as other NSAIDs—but importantly, there was a fourfold decrease of ulcers in patients who used Celebrex, in comparison to those who used nonselective NSAIDs. The FDA carefully examined all these results and approved Celebrex for the treatment of adults who suffer from osteoarthritis or rheumatoid arthritis.

Why do COX-2 inhibitors cause fewer gastrointestinal side effects than nonselective NSAIDs?

Because they are more selective in their actions, in many cases COX-2 inhibitors can control arthritis symptoms without causing stomach problems such as ulcers and bleeding.

Do COX-2 inhibitors completely eliminate the possibility of GI problems?

No. Although they reduce them significantly, COX-2 inhibitors cannot completely eliminate the possibility of side effects.

What does "COX" stand for?

COX is short for cyclooxygenase, an enzyme that helps make prostaglandins.

How do nonselective NSAIDs relieve arthritis pain?

They accomplish this by blocking the production of cyclooxygenase (or COX for short), an enzyme that helps make prostaglandins. Prostaglandins are the substances largely responsible for the pain and inflammation of arthritis.

So what's the problem with nonselective NSAIDs?

Scientists have discovered that there are two types of cyclooxygenase enzymes: COX 1 and COX 2. The COX 2 enzyme is linked to arthritis pain and inflammation, while the COX 1 enzyme—nicknamed "the housekeeping enzyme" because of its extremely useful functions in the body—protects the stomach lining and facilitates efficient platelet function.

Nonselective NSAIDs attack both the COX 1 and COX 2 enzymes. This means that they control pain and inflammation, but also disable the housekeeping COX 1 enzyme and prevent it from doing its jobs in protecting the body. By removing one important source of stomach protection, nonselective NSAIDs can unfortunately lead to ulcers and other gastrointestinal problems in susceptible individuals.

What makes COX-2 inhibitors different from the nonselective NSAIDs?

In therapeutic doses, more selective COX-2 inhibitors such as Celebrex and Vioxx block only the COX 2 enzyme responsible for arthritis pain and inflammation. They do not block the stomach-protective COX 1 enzyme. Therefore COX 1 goes on to help produce prostaglandins that protect the stomach from its own erosive acids.

What companies produce COX-2 inhibitors?

Celebrex is manufactured by G.D. Searle & Co., the pharmaceutical business unit of Monsanto. Vioxx is manufactured by Merck.

Are there any other COX-2 inhibitors?

Thus far Celebrex and Vioxx are the only FDA-approved COX-2 inhibitors, but more are on the way. The German company Boehringer Ingelheim GmbH expects to launch Mobic later this year. Mobic will be jointly marketed in the United States with Abbott Laboratories. Glaxo Wellcome of Great Britain, the second largest drug manufacturer in the world, also has a COX-2 inhibitor in development.

What other medications are used to ease the pain of arthritis?

They include:

• **Acetaminophen**, the aspirin-free alternative for people who are allergic to aspirin or have developed GI problems such as ulcers from aspirin or other NSAIDs. Acetaminophen provides pain relief but has no impact on swelling and inflammation.

- **Narcotics** to alleviate persistent, chronic pain. Doctors are cautious in prescribing drugs such as codeine and morphine because of their highly addictive nature.

- **Tranquilizers**, which soothe muscle tension. Because they are potentially addictive, tranquilizers should not be used for long periods of time.

- **Muscle relaxants**, which relieve pain by calming muscle spasms. Addictive like tranquilizers, muscle relaxants should only be used for short periods of time.

- **Antidepressants** to relieve chronic pain and promote sleep in people who suffer from problems such as fibromyalgia.

- **Nerve blocks**, which are injections of anesthetic directly into painful areas. Similar to the injection a dentist gives you before turning on the drill, nerve blocks are effective for short periods of time.

- **Cortisone shots**, which are injected directly into painful areas to reduce pain and swelling. Relief is longer lasting than with nerve blocks, but because of side effects injections must not be given too frequently.

- **Disease-modifying drugs**, or DMARDs, which reduce inflammation and slow the destructive process of inflammatory diseases like rheumatoid arthritis. They also help relieve pain.

- **Topical pain relievers** such as creams and lotions to provide temporary pain relief on painful areas.

PAIN-MANAGEMENT TECHNIQUES

Many pain-management techniques don't involve drugs at all. Arthritis sufferers also turn to techniques ranging from meditation and yoga to heat and cold treatments to relieve their aches and stiffness.

Create Your Own Plan for Pain Management

Because pain is a unique and individual experience, it's not surprising to learn that so is pain management. Certain strategies such as exercise and positive thinking are helpful for everyone, but other techniques you'll want to choose for yourself. For example, alternative approaches such as acupuncture or biofeedback work for some people but are not everyone's cup of tea. Work with your health-care team to develop a pain-management program that works for you. In addition to medication such as COX-2 inhibitors, your approach might contain some of the suggestions below.

Harness the Power of Positive Thinking

Accentuating the positive is essential when you have arthritis, for dwelling on pain only makes it seem worse. It's important to be firm and take control. When you feel helpless and depressed, pain is going to get the better of you rather than the other way around. Try to focus on positive thoughts, feelings, and actions instead of negative ones.

Give Yourself a Pep Talk

Counter negative feelings like anxiety, helplessness, and depression with positive self-encouragements. Prepare a few phrases and repeat them to yourself several times a day. Jot these phrases down on stick-on notes or index cards and put them on your bathroom mirror or bulletin board. Tuck cards in your briefcase or pocketbook.

For example, say:

"I am strong. I can handle this."

"It's better to feel pain than to feel nothing at all."

"Pain won't always be like this.
I'll feel better soon."

"There are people in much worse
situations than this."

"It's okay to rest. The world will not come to an
end if there are dishes in the sink."

"Exercises will make me feel better. If I keep doing
them, they'll get easier."

"Maybe I'll feel better tomorrow."

Keep a Journal

Putting your feelings and goals on paper can make you feel better. Later on, reviewing what you've written can help you gain a deeper perspective and come up with new solutions for old problems.

Maintain Your Sense of Humor

Humor is a potent antidote for pain.

Count Your Blessings

Focus on what you can do instead of what you can't do. Think about all the good things in your life—your family, your hobbies, your beautiful children or grandchildren.

Reward Yourself

Keep track of each positive step you take toward pain management and reward yourself for it. For example, after you do your stretching exercises, treat yourself to 10 minutes in the jacuzzi. In time, your victories will add up and you will gain increasing control over your pain.

Organize a Support System

The support of your family, friends, and health-care team is crucial to the management of pain and stress. Don't be afraid to reach out and ask for help when you need it. Asking for support—both emotional and physical—is better than becoming depressed, over-tired, or ill from trying to do too much.

Control Stress to Control Pain

Stress is the main trigger of Eastman Kodak retiree Laurie Stollery's aches and stiffness. She reaches out to others to help her control anxiety and keep things in perspective. "You need that support system," emphasizes Laurie, a participant in the Celebrex clinical trials. "My husband is my stabilizer. When I have his back-up and also my doctor's, I feel better. They help me remember that I'm doing all I can."

Don't Become Isolated

It's unwise to allow arthritis pain to isolate you from the rest of the world. Call a friend and schedule a date. When you spend too much time by yourself, you may find yourself trapped in the vicious pattern of pain you learned about earlier in this chapter. Remember, dwelling on physical limitations leads to depression, which leads to more pain, which leads to stress, which leads you right back to depression.

Share Your Feelings

Your family and friends care for you and don't want you to shut them out of what you are going through.

Ask for Help When You Need It

In addition to family and friends, consult your rabbi, priest, or minister. The Arthritis Foundation offers or can refer you to a wide variety of support groups and clubs, self-help courses, and aquatic and land-based exercise classes.

Join a Support Group

Share your feelings and frustrations with people who face similar problems and concerns. In a support group you'll learn more about your disease and new ways to cope with it. To locate a group in your area, contact your local branch of the Arthritis Foundation.

Surf the Net

When stiffness and pain kept arthritis sufferer Laurie Schuster from getting to the library, she got an Internet connection. On-line access gets cheaper and easier to use every day, and a chat room with others who suffer from arthritis can function as your on-line support group.

Relax Your Body and Mind

When you are in pain, you are under physical and emotional stress. Pain and stress have similar impacts on your body. Both lead to rapid breathing, tense muscles, and elevated heart rate and blood pressure. Relaxation methods can help you control stress, manage pain, and recapture your overall sense of well-being. (Read more about these methods in Chapter Ten.)

Say a Prayer

Attend a service at your church or temple, for prayer can have a remarkably powerful healing influence. If you can't get out of the house, inspirational tapes are available.

Meditate

Meditation requires concentration that helps to block out pain. There are many different types of meditation. One method is to sit quietly and repeat in your head a certain word or mantra such as "peace" or "Om." You can also meditate by visualizing a calm image like waves rolling onto a beach, or by focusing on your breathing.

Practice Guided Imagery

Close your eyes and relax. Picture yourself in a safe and happy place. Imagine all its sights, sounds, and colors, and all the different ways in which it affects your senses. This will take your focus off pain.

Try Hypnosis

See a psychologist or counselor if you want to test this method of pain management, which combines deep meditation and guided imagery.

Listen to Relaxation Tapes

Many tapes can take you step by step through the process of deep relaxation. Others feature soothing sounds such as rain falling, whales calling, or leaves rustling in the wind. Of course, be it Bach or Sinatra or Lauryn Hill, you might find your own favorite music most relaxing of all.

Make Healthy Lifestyle Choices

A healthy lifestyle can't cure your arthritis, but it can go a long way to help you feel stronger overall and better equipped to face the challenges of your disease.

Eat a Balanced Diet

Especially when you are experiencing a flare, you may be tempted to neglect your diet. Appetite fades, and the thought of getting out to the store with aching legs or preparing a meal with stiff fingers may seem like more trouble than it is worth. You may be tempted to turn to comfort foods like salty chips and dips or pints of creamy ice cream. But these are high in fat and sugar and empty in nutrients, and will only increase your fatigue and further aggravate your condition. Even when you are feeling under the weather, make an effort to eat healthy foods.

Avoid Alcohol and Drugs

Don't fall into the trap of trying to control arthritis pain with alcohol or illegal drugs. Dangerous and addictive, these substances will only worsen your health problems. If you are taking medication for arthritis, there can be hazardous interactions.

Get a Good Night's Sleep

If you're not getting enough sleep, you're opening the door to pain and stress. In addition to giving your joints a rest to reduce pain and swelling, sleep affords you the energy to cope with your arthritis on a daily basis. (Turn to Chapter Nine for specific tips on how to get a good night's sleep.)

Practice Joint-Saving Strategies

Joint protection is an important part of pain management. See a physical or occupational therapist for advice on how to go about day-to-day activities in ways that reduce the stress on painful joints. For example, use your strongest joints and muscle groups to lift objects.

Use Braces and Splints as Necessary

By stabilizing joints, orthotic devices such as these reduce pain and inflammation.

Learn to Respect Your Pain

If your joints hurt for more than two hours after exercise or activity, you've done too much. Next time ease up and do a little less.

Get Regular Exercise

Exercise is beneficial to pain management in many ways. Stretching or range-of-motion (ROM) exercises can help you continue to move your joints in as painless a way as possible. Aerobic activity such as walking and biking stimulates the release of endorphins, your body's natural painkillers. Strengthening exercises can keep bone and cartilage strong, which provides more stability for weakened or damaged joints. Finally, regular exercise can help you control pain, stress, and anxiety and allow you to get a good night's sleep.

Balance Exercise with Rest

If activities that you regularly did before now cause you pain, don't force yourself to do them. You may injure yourself and cause further inflammation or tissue damage.

Do Your ROM Exercises Every Day

Find the time to practice ROM exercises once or twice every day. These gentle stretches are your best bet to reduce stiffness and pain and keep joints flexible. See Chapter Eight for more information on ROM exercises.

Try Yoga or Tai Chi

The relaxing postures of yoga or tai chi may prove especially beneficial. In addition to increasing your range of motion, they noticeably reduce stress and tension.

After the Workout

After your swim or stretch, treat yourself to a relaxing visit to the sauna, steam room, or whirlpool. Heat is especially soothing to stiff and aching joints. Have a massage to increase blood circulation, smoothe out muscle knots, and relieve pain.

Use Heat and Cold Treatments

Heat and cold treatments are very helpful in the relief of arthritis pain. Use whichever works best for you, or alternate heat and cold. Heat treatments ranging from hot water bottles to jacuzzis are good for your circulation and relax your muscles, while cold numbs painful areas and reduces swelling.

Thermotherapy

Heat treatments should be comfortably warm, but not too hot. Hot, moist compresses or towels, commercial hot packs, hot water bottles, heating pads, heat lamps, and hot baths and showers can all act as effective heat applications. Incorporate thermotherapy in regular visits to your gym by swimming in the heated pool and relaxing in the steam room, sauna, or jacuzzi.

Cryotherapy

Numbing cold can slow down nerve activity and thus reduce the pain and swelling of arthritis. If you don't have an ice pack, just put a few ice cubes in a plastic bag or take a package of frozen vegetables and place it on the painful area. If you have recurrent arthritis pain, invest in a reusable commercial cold pack from your local drugstore and store it in the freezer. Wrap ice in a towel and be careful not to leave it on the skin for too long. If your skin grows numb, remove the ice to avoid frostbite.

Pace Yourself

Don't cause yourself further pain and stress by trying to squeeze too much into your day:

- Schedule your activities carefully so you don't expend excess energy.

- Eliminate unnecessary errands. Patronize restaurants, grocery stores, and pharmacies that deliver.

- Shop by catalog.

- Go to the full-service island at your gas station.

- When you're already feeling that you have more than you can handle, don't be afraid to say no when a family member or friend asks you to make an extra trip or run one more errand.

- Familiarize yourself with the Internet. It's amazing how much you can do on line these days. You can even order your groceries via computer.

- Stay up to date with technology. Instead of trying to make your way to the post office, e-mail your work in.

- Arrange for your phone and electric bills to be automatically paid from your checking account each month.

- Have your paycheck or Social Security check automatically deposited in your bank account.

- Break each task into manageable parts. In that way, it won't appear to be so overwhelming.

- Use self-help devices such as large-handled utensils for eating, grab bars for bathroom use, lever faucet and tap turners, electric can openers, zipper pulls, buttoning aids, reach extenders, and electric garage door openers.

- Think of more creative ways to make living with arthritis easier.

Try an Alternative Treatment

While most people control arthritis with medication such as COX-2 inhibitors and standard pain management techniques, some turn to alternatives such as acupuncture or herbal remedies. (Read more about these alternatives in Chapter Ten.)

WHEN SURGERY IS NECESSARY

Fortunately, most people who have arthritis will never need joint surgery. A well-balanced program of medication and self-help strategies such as exercise, rest, physical therapy, and joint protection is usually successful in managing aches, stiffness, and inflammation. But when arthritis fails to respond to these measures, surgery may be the only way to repair joints and control symptoms.

In what circumstances is surgery necessary?

* When persistent or severe pain fails to respond to other treatment

* When pain is so disabling that it interferes with day-to-day activities

* When your range of motion is so severely limited that you cannot move your knee to walk or your arm to dress yourself

* When joint damage is severe and progressive

* When joints become crippled or misshapen with arthritis

What are the benefits of surgery for arthritis?

The most dramatic benefit is pain relief. If your joints were not too severely damaged going into surgery, you may also recover use of your joints and increased range of motion.

What are the risks associated with surgery?

There are risks associated with any surgery, especially if you are elderly or in poor health. If you are to undergo general rather than local anesthesia, your physician needs to make sure that your heart and lungs are strong enough.

How do I know if surgery is right for me?

Your doctor will help you make the right decision based on your condition and a careful analysis of the risks and benefits. If you're still not sure, by all means get a second opinion from another physician.

What is the best way to prepare for surgery?

The better shape your body is in going in to surgery, the better the prognosis. When possible, try to ready yourself with strengthening exercises and physical therapy. A well-balanced diet is also a must. To prepare yourself emotionally, learn all you can about what to expect before, during, and after surgery.

Is it okay to keep taking NSAIDs before surgery?

This is a question to address with your doctor, because nonselective NSAIDs affect blood clotting. Ask your doctor whether COX-2 inhibitors might be a wiser choice at this time.

What types of surgery are available for arthritis?

They include:

- **Arthroscopy,** a minimally invasive surgical procedure in which a surgeon repairs a joint through a small incision. It is often performed on the knee, and usually doesn't even require an overnight stay in the hospital.

- **Bone fusion,** a surgical procedure that fuses together two bones forming a joint to provide greater strength and stability.

- **Osteotomy,** in which bone is cut and repositioned in order to correct a deformity.

- **Resection,** a surgical procedure in which all or part of a bone is removed to improve function and relieve pain.

- **Synovectomy,** in which diseased synovium (joint lining) is removed. This reduces pain and swelling, and can slow or prevent further damage.

- **Total joint replacement,** a surgical procedure in which severely damaged joints (most commonly hips and knees) are replaced with artificial joints made of flexible material like plastic.

What is the recovery period from surgery like?

This depends on the type of surgery. In general, your doctor will prescribe a combination of rest, joint protection, and physical therapy. You may have to rest for days or weeks before resuming your normal routine. Even then, your activity will probably be more limited than usual. For a time, you may need the assistance of a brace, splint, cane, walker, or wheelchair. An occupational therapist can show you how to safely move your joints as you go about your day-to-day activities. When you are ready, it's time to begin physical therapy.

What is the reason for physical therapy following surgery?

Physical therapy will help you regain use of your joints and muscles. Although this is hard work and there is pain in moving stiff muscles and joints, in the long run the rewards are greater function and less pain.

Why is physical therapy sometimes difficult and painful?

After surgery, when the swelling goes down, the new or repaired joint should be less stiff. However, the muscles around the joint are just as weak or even weaker than before. In addition, tendons and ligaments that surround a joint and hold it in place may be weak and stiff from misuse or disuse.

The exercises your physical therapist performs with you will strengthen the tissues supporting your joints. Over time, the exercises themselves will grow less painful. And most importantly, you will gain greater range of motion and experience less pain overall.

PART III

NATURAL TREATMENTS FOR ARTHRITIS

SEVEN

◆◆◆

Diet and Arthritis

Last night I had calamari fra diavolo for dinner, and it was delicious. I would have been afraid to order anything like that before I started taking Celebrex.

Laurie Schuster, 37-year-old osteoarthritis patient and participant in Celebrex clinical trials

Good diet and nutrition play a part in preventing and controlling all types of diseases, and scientists today are investigating exactly what role they play in arthritis. So far we know that diet has a direct impact on gout and osteoporosis, and weight control is an important part of arthritis management. On the other hand, diet does not cause arthritis and there are no magic foods that you can eat to cure this disease. In addition, if you are taking certain medications for your arthritis, you will have to watch what you eat.

GOUT

What is the relationship between gout and diet?

People who have gout have an excess amount of uric acid in their blood. Uric acid is a waste product of purines, which are compounds found in rich foods like organ meats and fish such as sardines, herring, and mussels. If you have gout, your doctor will probably recommend that you eat purine-rich foods in moderation only. Weight control is also an important part of managing this disease, since being overweight increases your body's production of uric acid.

What foods are rich in purines?

Foods with a high purine or uric acid content include:

- Very high: organ meats, herring, herring roe, mussels, sardines, smelts, yeast

- High: anchovies, bacon, cod, goose, haddock, liver, kidneys, mackerel, pheasant, salmon, scallops, trout, turkey, veal, venison

- Moderately high: asparagus, bass, beef, bouillon, chicken, crab, duck, eel, halibut, ham, kidney beans, lentils, liverwurst, lobster, mushrooms, navy beans, oysters, peas, pork, shrimp, spinach, tripe

I've heard that drinking red wine can aggravate gout. Is this true?

Yes. Alcohol can trigger gout attacks, as can being overweight and having high blood pressure. If you suffer from this disease, your doctor will probably recommend that you have only one or two drinks a week, or abstain from alcohol altogether.

OSTEOPOROSIS

What is the relationship between osteoporosis and diet?

A diet rich in calcium, along with regular weight-bearing exercise, can help reduce your risk of developing this potentially very serious bone-thinning, arthritis-related disease.

Why is calcium important?

Calcium builds strong bones in your youth and slows bone loss in your middle and later years.

What can I do to help prevent osteoporosis?

Women, who are at a greater risk for this disease than men, should consider adding several glasses of calcium-packed low-fat milk to their diets today in order to prevent the ravages of osteoporosis in later life.

Does skim milk have as much calcium as whole milk?

Yes. Each has about 300 milligrams per 8-ounce glass. Nonfat dairy products are just as good sources of calcium as their richer counterparts, and are healthier choices overall.

How much calcium should I include in my diet to prevent bone loss?

For young women, a healthy diet includes 1,200 milligrams of calcium and 400 international units of vitamin D each day. After menopause, when estrogen levels plummet, women should increase their calcium intake to 1,500 milligrams a day.

I'm only in my thirties. Do I really need to start thinking about osteoporosis now?

Unquestionably, it is at menopause (the final menstrual period) that women face a sudden and precipitous rise in their risk of osteoporosis. But because we begin storing calcium in our bones at a young age, it's never too early to start strengthening them with diet and exercise.

I'm lactose intolerant. Are there any other good dietary sources of calcium?

While dairy products such as low-fat or nonfat milk, cheese, and yogurt are the best source of this mineral, you can also get calcium from eating leafy green and yellow vegetables, canned sardines and salmon (including the ground bones), seeds, nuts, soy foods, and fortified cereals and juices. Lactose-reduced milk and other dairy products are also available.

What about calcium supplements?

These are another option. If you can't get enough calcium in your diet, ask your doctor to recommend a supplement. Be sure to take one that also contains vitamin D.

Why is vitamin D important for strong bones?

Vitamin D is necessary to help your body effectively absorb calcium. Spending as little as 15 minutes in the sun each week without wearing sunblock will provide all the vitamin D you need. Alternatively, if you're concerned about sun damage choose cereals and milk fortified with vitamin D.

I've heard that some foods prevent our bodies from making the best use of calcium. Is this true?

Yes. Substances such as caffeine, alcohol, sugar, and red meat can indeed hamper your body's ability to absorb calcium. Because high-protein diets actually pull or leach calcium from the bones, vegetarians pack extra natural protection against osteoporosis.

WEIGHT MANAGEMENT

Is controlling my weight an important part of arthritis management?

Yes. Being either overweight or underweight can be a problem if you have or are at risk of developing arthritis:

- Being overweight puts you at a greater risk of osteoarthritis, particularly in weight-bearing joints such as the knees, hips, ankles, and feet. If you already have arthritis, excess weight puts extra strain on your joints and can worsen your degree of disability.

- On the other hand, being underweight can also be a problem. During a flare of rheumatoid arthritis, your appetite fades and you may lose weight. But it's very important to keep your strength up when you suffer from a chronic disease. Try to make it a point to eat regular, healthy meals even during these difficult periods.

Why is being overweight a risk factor for osteoarthritis?

There are a number of reasons for this. Excess weight means excess stress on weight-bearing joints such as your hips, knees, and feet. If you are susceptible to OA but have not yet developed it, being overweight can tip the scales over into the danger zone. If your joints are already affected with arthritis, they may grow worse. In addition, when you are both obese and arthritic, you may find that it takes longer to move around and get enough exercise to shed excess pounds. Fat may also prevent medication from traveling to affected joints as efficiently.

If I have osteoarthritis, how much weight do I have to lose?

That depends on your height, weight, and type of body frame. But if you and your doctor determine that you are overweight, now's the time to shed those excess pounds. The good news is that losing as little as 10 or 11 pounds can cut your risk of developing osteoarthritis. Talk to your physician about developing safe, healthy, and realistic weight-loss goals. Keep in mind that not only will losing weight improve joint pain and stiffness, it will also help you feel better overall, psychologically as well as physically.

In addition to my doctor, are there any other health care professionals who can help me lose weight?

A nutritionist or registered dietician can help you design a sensible weight-loss program. It's important to make sure that you continue to consume enough nutrients while you lose weight, and a medical professional can help you accomplish this.

What is the difference between a nutritionist and a registered dietician?

A registered dietician (or RD for short) is certified by the American Dietctic Association (ADA). Certification comes with graduation from an accredited four-year college with a degree in nutrition; participation in an ADA-approved internship; successful completion of a qualifying examination; and continuing education. Although no special training or certification is required for nutritionists, there are some very good ones out there.

How do I find a good nutritionist or dietician?

Your doctor can refer you to a qualified nutritionist or dietician. Word of mouth is also helpful, so talk to friends who have successfully lost weight. Or you may choose to join a support group via your local chapter of the Arthritis Foundation and ask other members for helpful names and numbers.

My friend lost weight on a liquid diet and suggested I try it. Is this a good idea?

No. Chances are that very soon your friend will regain the pounds she lost on that diet. The only sensible way to lose weight and to keep it off is to eat less and exercise more. Over time, this will lead to a more gradual, healthier, and longer-lasting weight loss.

What about dieter's teas? Are these a safe bet?

No. These teas usually contain laxative herbs such as senna, aloe, cascara, or rhubarb root. Temporary weight loss comes via diarrhea and dehydration, a very dangerous route. In the early 1990s, several young women died after extended periods of drinking senna tea.

What's the problem with fad diets?

Fad diets are not a good idea for anyone, but they can be especially dangerous for people who suffer from chronic diseases like arthritis. A very low-calorie or liquid diet can leave you feeling tired and worn out, and it deprives you of necessary nutrients. If you're trying to lose weight, always avoid radical and restricted fad or crash diets that can lead quickly to unsafe nutrient deficiencies.

What is the safest way to lose weight?

A diet low in fat and calories and high in fiber-rich whole foods, in combination with regular aerobic exercise, is the safest long-term formula for weight loss.

How do I know what type of exercise program is right for me?

This depends on what type of arthritis you have, its severity, and what joints are affected. A doctor or therapist can help you figure out the exercise program that is best for you.

How often do I need to exercise to lose weight? And for how long?

Significant health benefits kick in when you do aerobic exercises at least three times a week for 30 minutes. But remember: Begin slowly. If you've been inactive, don't try to do this all at once. For example, start out walking just five or 10 minutes at a time. Gradually increase the length of your workouts, and when you reach 20 minutes pick up your cruising speed.

Can you give me an example of a healthy weight-loss plan?

A healthy diet on which you can shed a few pounds includes lots of fresh fruits, whole grains, and vegetables, accompanied by small portions of meat and fish. Dairy products should be fat-free, and saturated fats kept to an absolute minimum. Consult with your doctor or nutritionist to develop a weight-loss plan that will work best for you.

I have rheumatoid arthritis. Should I be concerned about my weight?

If you have RA, you should probably be more worried about losing rather than gaining weight. During flares, getting to the store, shopping, preparing a meal, and cleaning up afterward may seem like an enormous effort. It can even seem like more trouble than it's worth. Still, when you lose your appetite during these painful periods, it's important to eat sensibly and maintain your normal weight. Now's the time to turn to those convenience foods, perhaps with the addition of a healthy salad and fresh fruit for dessert. On the other hand, if your doctor does prescribe corticosteroids to control rheumatoid arthritis, ask about dietary recommendations to avoid weight gain, a common side effect of these medications.

A HEALTHY DIET

What are the basic elements of a healthy diet?

In 1992 the United States Department of Agriculture and Health and Human Services devised the Food Guide Pyramid to illustrate basic good eating habits. They recommended the following food groups and number of servings of each to be consumed by healthy adults on a daily basis:

- 6 to 11 servings of bread, cereal, rice, and pasta

- 3 to 5 servings of vegetables

- 2 to 4 servings of fruits

- 2 to 3 servings of proteins (meat, poultry, fish, dried beans, eggs, and nuts)

- 2 to 3 servings of dairy foods

- Only small amounts of fats, oils, and sweets

But I have arthritis. What is the best diet for me?

Your best bet in controlling chronic health problems like arthritis is a whole foods diet rich in vegetables and fiber and low in animal fat, salt, sugar, refined carbohydrates, and alcohol. Depending on your specific health needs and which medications you are taking, your doctor may also make specific dietary recommendations or refer you to a registered dietician or nutritionist. Following are some general guidelines for a healthy diet:

- **Eat a variety of foods.** Chronic illness and the medications prescribed to treat them can rob your body of valuable nutrients. To make sure your body gets all the vitamins and minerals it needs, consume a variety of foods from all different categories: green leafy, orange, red, and yellow vegetables; fruits rich in vitamin C and other nutrients; whole grains; lean meats and seafood; dried beans; and low-fat or nonfat milk, cheese, yogurt, and other dairy products.

- **Maintain a healthy weight.** Being either overweight or underweight can aggravate arthritis symptoms.

- **Use saturated fats and cholesterol in moderate amounts only.** Nutritional guidelines recommend that no more than 30% of your daily calories come from fat, but many experts stress that 20% or even less is best. So tonight, think lean and low-fat. Instead of a cheeseburger, grab a turkey burger, a vegetable burger, or a tuna salad made with low-fat mayonnaise for dinner. If you choose to eat meat, limit yourself to a 3-ounce portion— about the size of a deck of cards.

- **Eat plenty of fresh fruits, vegetables, and whole grains.** Foods that are rich in complex carbohydrates provide valuable nutrition and are also an excellent source of fiber, which can prevent the constipation associated with some arthritis medications. Eat plenty of fresh fruits (flavonoid-packed berries are considered especially good for arthritis), vegetables, and whole grains and cereals like wheat bran and brown rice.

- **Limit your intake of sugar and alcohol.** The empty calories in sugary sweets and alcohol can inflate your weight without providing any nutritional value. Cakes and doughnuts provide a quick sugar rush—and then as quickly a crash which can leave you feeling extra vulnerable to pain and fatigue. Alcohol can trigger a gout attack, interfere with arthritis medications, and leave you feeling befuddled and unable to cope with your condition.

- **Cut back on salt and sodium-packed processed and fast foods.** Salt or sodium causes you to retain water and can inflate your blood pressure. Uncomfortable water retention and bloating are already a side effect of certain arthritis medications (particularly corticosteroids), while high blood pressure can trigger an attack of gout.

- **Make sure you consume the recommended daily allowances of vitamins and minerals such as calcium and vitamin D.** When in doubt, the surest way to do this is to take a good daily multivitamin.

- **Drink eight glasses of water every day.** Pure water flushes harmful toxins from your body and keeps you from becoming dehydrated or constipated.

Exactly what are nutrients, anyway?

These are the substances in foods that are necessary for the proper functioning of our bodies and the many complex chemical reactions taking place in them.

Is a daily multivitamin a good idea?

Yes. Even with an excellent diet it is difficult to take in all the nutrients we need on a daily basis. In addition, the nutrient needs of people who have arthritis are increased due to stress, pain, fatigue, and the environmental toxins to which we are all routinely subjected in our day-to-day lives.

What kinds of fruits are best?

Whole fresh fruits are richest in fiber as well as nutrients, and are preferable to juice. If you choose canned or frozen fruit, avoid products with added sugars and syrup.

What role does fiber play in the body?

Fiber is essential in preventing constipation and resultant complications such as diverticulosis, diverticulitis, and irritable bowel syndrome. Fiber can also help you control cholesterol and maintain normal blood sugar levels.

What kinds of vegetables are best?

The more colorful your dinner, the healthier it is. This is because richly colored vegetables are also richest in valuable nutrients. Yellow-orange fruits and vegetables are packed with antioxidants, which may help relieve arthritis inflammation. Dark green leafy vegetables like spinach, mustard greens, and turnip greens provide potent anticancer protection.

Is it possible to consume too many nutrients?

If you're talking about nutrients from food sources alone, it's highly unlikely. But if you're taking vitamin supplements in excess of recommended daily allowances, or RDAs, be sure to consult with your doctor. Excess nutrients in supplement form can lead to problems such as ulcers. The fat-soluble A, D, E, and K vitamins can lead to serious disease when taken in excess.

I've heard that fish oils can be beneficial. Is this true?

Research does suggest that the oils from cold-water fish may be helpful in controlling arthritis. This is because cold-water fish such as salmon, mackerel, sardines, and cod are packed with omega-3 fatty acids.

What are omega-3 fatty acids?

These are the "good fats." Omega-3 unsaturated fatty acids such as eicosapentaenoic acid (EPA) and docosahexaenoic acid (DHA) in certain fish are naturally anti-inflammatory and can also give the immune systems of RA sufferers a boost.

To receive significant health benefits, how often should I eat fish?

Eat fish two or three times a week. Beyond the specific health benefits vis-à-vis arthritis, fish are a better choice overall than fat-laden cheeseburgers or processed meats.

What are some good food sources of omega-3 fatty acids?

These include:
Anchovies
Bluefish
Cod
Herring
Mackerel
Sablefish
Salmon
Sardines
Smelt

Swordfish
Trout
Tuna

I'm not much of a fish eater. Is there any other way to supplement my diet with omega-3 fatty acids?

A teaspoon or two of fish oil each day may be helpful. Be careful to take no more than this, for too much fish oil can cause problems with blood clotting.

Is it also beneficial to eat foods rich in antioxidants?

Yes. Antioxidants can neutralize some of the free radicals released during joint inflammation, and research has suggested that people who have osteoarthritis are deficient in these valuable nutrients. While no single food can cure arthritis, a diet rich in antioxidants may ease some of your symptoms and will make you feel better overall.

What are free radicals?

Cell-damaging free radicals are by-products of inflammation and the processing of oxygen in the body. Free radical formation is also boosted by environmental variables such as infection, smoking, air pollution, and too much exposure to the sun.

Can you name some antioxidants with which I might be familiar?

Antioxidants include vitamin A, carotenoids (the plant form of vitamin A), vitamin C, vitamin E, and selenium.

Is betacarotene an antioxidant?

Yes. But while betacarotene is the most well-known carotenoid, it is far from the only one. There are actually many different carotenoids present in fruits and vegetables.

What foods are good sources of antioxidants?

Following are some excellent sources:

- **Carotenoids:** yellow-orange fruits and vegetables such as cantaloupe, peaches, papayas, mangoes, sweet potatoes, yams, and carrots; dark green leafy vegetables like broccoli, spinach, and all kinds of greens (turnip, mustard, etc.)

- **Vitamin A:** turkey, milk, and liver

- **Vitamin C:** fresh fruits such as oranges, grapefruit, kiwi, papayas, mangoes, bananas, and strawberries; fresh vegetables, including asparagus, broccoli, cabbage, greens, potatoes, and red peppers (because vitamin C is destroyed in cooking, eat vegetables lightly steamed)

- **Vitamin E:** whole-grain breads and cereals, sunflower seeds, flaxseed and sunflower oil, avocadoes, nuts, and wheat germ

- **Selenium:** swordfish, salmon, tuna, shrimp, and oysters

What about antioxidant vitamins?

Whole foods are the best source of antioxidants, but if you can't manage to get enough antioxidants in your regular diet ask your doctor about prescribing or recommending a supplement.

I've heard that bioflavonoids can be helpful too. Is this true?

Yes. Bioflavonoids found in plant foods prevent collagen (an essential part of cartilage) from deteriorating. And like antioxidants, they can also prevent free radical damage.

What are good sources of bioflavonoids?

Green tea and all kinds of berries (blueberries, strawberries, raspberries, and blackberries) are excellent sources of bioflavonoids. Additional sources include other fresh fruits, vegetables, whole grains, and seeds.

What about organic foods?

Again, they're no cure for arthritis, but organic foods are certainly a healthy addition to your diet.

Organically grown fruits and vegetables are free of the potentially harmful chemicals used to grow, store, preserve, and ship most commercial produce. Organic animal products are also important, so that we can avoid the consumption of excess estrogen, growth hormones, and antibiotics that are routinely given to farm animals to increase their meat and milk production.

Are food additives safe?

While there's no clear correlation with arthritis, food additives such as colors, flavors, and preservatives cause adverse reactions in some people. If you suspect that these are linked to arthritis flares, there's clearly no harm in eliminating them from your diet.

Is it safe for me to drink alcohol if I have arthritis?

Alcohol has many troublesome effects on your health and should be strictly avoided with certain medications. If you are taking NSAIDs in combination with alcohol, gastrointestinal side effects can be worse. Combining alcohol with the arthritis medications acetaminophen or methotrexate can lead to liver damage. In addition, alcohol can increase the level of uric acid in your blood and lead to an attack of gout. Its empty calories lead to excess pounds.

Is there any special diet I can follow to get rid of arthritis?

Unfortunately, no. Out of desperation and frustration, many arthritis sufferers turn to crazy diets with this or that megadose of vitamins and minerals. But there is no one "ideal" diet to cure arthritis, as nutritional needs vary from individual to individual. Beware of false promises of magic cures.

I'm confused by all the different recommendations of vitamins and minerals for arthritis. Is there anyone who can help me sort through them and determine which ones are right for me?

In addition to your doctor, a nutritionist or a registered dietician can help you sort through the various choices, design a healthy diet, and select which (if any) supplements are appropriate for you. Ask your doctor for a referral.

FOOD ALLERGIES

Do food allergies play a role in arthritis?

The role of food allergies in arthritis has long been a controversial one. The bottom line appears to be that in a small number of people, food allergies may indeed aggravate the symptoms of rheumatoid arthritis. But although allergies may trigger a flare, they do not cause arthritis, and eliminating allergens from your diet will not cure you of arthritis.

What are some common food allergens?

They include:

- Wheat
- Corn
- Dairy products
- Shellfish
- Food additives
- Citrus fruits

What should I do if I think food allergies are aggravating my arthritis and triggering flares?

If you suspect that an allergy to milk or wheat or corn or shellfish is causing arthritis flares, work with your doctor or a nutritionist to identify and eliminate from your diet those foods to which you are sensitive or allergic. Even though doing this will not cure your arthritis, by reducing flares it will make you feel better overall.

How can I determine if foods are triggering my symptoms?

One helpful strategy is to keep a journal of all the foods you eat along with incidents of joint pain and inflammation. If you notice that your arthritis flares up when you eat certain foods, see if eliminating them from your diet for a time brings significant improvement.

What is an elimination diet?

Some rheumatoid arthritis sufferers turn to elimination diets in order to determine if allergies are triggering their symptoms. These diets involve eliminating suspected allergens from the diet for several days or weeks, and then reintroducing them one by one. But beware: Elimination diets can rob your body of necessary nutrients.

What is the safest way to try an elimination diet?

These diets should only be undertaken under the careful guidance of your doctor or nutritionist.

I've heard that avoiding eggplant and tomatoes can be helpful. Is this true?

Natural practitioners sometimes recommend that rheumatoid arthritis sufferers should avoid these and other nightshade vegetables (which also include white potatoes, peppers, and squash). These members of the nightshade family contain chemicals called solanines, to which RA sufferers may be sensitive. Although there is little hard scientific evidence to support these claims, a number of people have found relief by avoiding these foods.

Does fasting have any impact on arthritis?

Short-term fasting, or abstaining from food, has proven helpful to some RA sufferers. However, fast-

ing should always take place under the careful guidance of your doctor or nutritionist. Fasting for more
than a short period of time can damage your heart and
other body systems.

What about a vegetarian diet? Is that helpful?

As with fasting, some arthritis sufferers feel better
when they follow a low-fat vegetarian diet. This may
be because arachidonic acid, a fatty acid in animal
foods, provokes joint inflammation. In addition, a diet
revolving around meat may emphasize phosphorus
rather than calcium, which causes calcium to leach out
of the bones. This in turn may lead to calcium de-
posits around the joints, a common problem in people
who have osteoarthritis.

What is the safest way to try a vegetarian diet?

If you'd like to try a vegetarian diet, tell your doctor of your plans and be sure that you still take in
enough protein by consuming plenty of beans and
grains.

DIET AND ARTHRITIS MEDICATIONS

Is there any special time that I should take my arthritis medication? Should I take it on an empty stomach or with meals?

This is a good question to ask your doctor, for the
answer depends upon the particular medication you

are taking. To avoid stomach upset, it's a good idea to take nonsteroidal anti-inflammatory drugs (NSAIDs) with food, a glass of milk, or an antacid. On the other hand, if you are taking medications such as methotrexate or penicillamine for rheumatoid arthritis, it's best to take them on an empty stomach. Again, always be sure to ask your doctor or pharmacist about any special instructions for taking drugs.

Does taking NSAIDs with meals really help?

It definitely helps to take NSAIDs with meals, or even with just a cracker or a glass of milk. Don't attempt to take them on an empty stomach. "That stuff will tear your stomach up if you don't eat with it," says Celebrex clinical study participant Laurie Schuster of the NSAIDs she used to take for her osteoarthritis.

What should I do if arthritis medications continue to upset my stomach? Is it true that switching from nonselective NSAIDs to COX-2 inhibitors may alleviate stomach discomfort?

This may be a helpful strategy for you. For example, Laurie successfully brought her stomach problems to a close when she began taking Celebrex. If gastrointestinal effects such as bleeding or ulcers continue to be a problem for you despite taking NSAIDs with meals, ask your doctor about the new COX-2 inhibitors. In clinical trials, therapeutic amounts of

COX-2 inhibitors were associated with fewer gastro-intestinal problems.

What impact can arthritis medications have on my nutritional status?

Medications have many unintentional side effects on your body. For example, some anti-arthritis drugs can affect the liver and kidneys, and this in turn can have an impact on how your body absorbs and utilizes valuable nutrients. NSAIDs irritate the stomach lining, and some can lower the level of vitamin C in your body. Antacids that you take to relieve stomach irritation often contain aluminum and magnesium, which can decrease your absorption of phosphorus. The bottom line is that taking drugs—especially for long periods of time—can deplete your body of valuable nutrients.

Are there any actions I can take to offset the nutritional side effects of medications?

Absolutely. This varies, of course, on a case by case basis according to the medication you are taking. We provide a few examples here, but the impact that each drug has on your body is unique and sometimes extensive. Your best bet is to consult your doctor or pharmacist for in-depth information and advice.

I'm taking NSAIDs. Will this have any nutritional effect on my body?

Yes. Some NSAIDs can decrease your absorption of vitamin C, a valuable antioxidant. You can counteract this effect by eating vitamin C–packed oranges, grapefruit, and red peppers.

My stomach is so upset from NSAIDs that I can't keep my food down. What can I do?

Taking NSAIDs with food is the best way to prevent them from causing stomach upset. If this doesn't prove sufficient, ask your doctor about switching to new COX-2 inhibitors such as Celebrex or Vioxx.

I need to take antacids with NSAIDs, because otherwise my stomach gets upset. Are there any foods I can eat to counteract their effects on my body?

Because antacids may interfere with your absorption of phosphorus, eat an extra serving each day of phosphorus-rich foods such as milk, fish, poultry, eggs, milk, soybeans, or peanut butter.

I'm taking methotrexate for my rheumatoid arthritis. Should I be concerned about its impact on my nutritional status?

Yes. Methotrexate may interfere with your absorption of folic acid.

Why is folic acid important?

Folic acid is a B vitamin that can help lower levels of homocysteine, a substance that increases your risk of heart disease. It also helps prevent birth defects. The recommended daily allowance is 400 micrograms.

What are good food sources of folic acid?

Beans are a good source of folic acid, as are cereals enriched with B vitamins like folic acid and B_{12}. When in doubt, check the labels in your local supermarket. If you find that you are not getting enough folic acid in your regular diet, ask your physician about prescribing or recommending a supplement.

What about corticosteroids?

Corticosteroids have many uncomfortable and sometimes even dangerous side effects. Although they effectively relieve inflammation, because of their many adverse effects on the body these drugs should always be used with circumspection.

I've put on weight and feel bloated and uncomfortable since I began taking corticosteroids. Can I stop taking them?

No. One thing you should *never* do is stop taking these or any other prescribed medications on your own. If the side effects grow intolerable, ask your doctor about reducing your dosage and/or changing your medication.

Why do medication changes require such close medical supervision?

It is dangerous to suddenly stop or reduce your dosage of corticosteroids. This may lead to a sudden flare of symptoms or other problems. While it is true that they have unpleasant and sometimes even dangerous side effects such as fluid retention, weight gain, and high blood pressure, corticosteroids can be very effective tools in the management of arthritis. Only your doctor can accurately assess their risks versus benefits. However, be sure to openly and honestly discuss your concerns with your physician, and ask about any possible alternatives.

Are there any measures I can take to counteract the side effects of corticosteroids?

Because they make you more susceptible to osteoporosis, when you take corticosteroids for any significant length of time your doctor should carefully monitor your bone density. A good calcium and vitamin D supplement is a must. And while all arthritis sufferers should follow a healthy diet, this is especially important if you are taking corticosteroids.

What can I do to control the effects of arthritis medications on my diet and nutrition?

Educating yourself about arthritis drugs and their side effects is your best bet. When you know what to expect, you can take actions such as making dietary

adjustments or taking vitamin and mineral supplements to offset potential side effects. Be sure to ask
your doctor or pharmacist about the possible side effects of all drugs that you take for your arthritis.

EIGHT
◆◆◆

The Anti-Arthritis Exercise Program

The more active I keep my body, the better I feel. I walk six miles a week and ride my bike too. When my joints are stiff and my muscles are sore, soaking in our jacuzzi always helps. And if I get tired, I just take a rest. It's okay to fall asleep for an hour.

Laurie Stollery, 60-year-old osteoarthritis patient and participant in Celebrex clinical trials

A proper balance of exercise and rest can go a long way toward keeping you healthy and energized. Exercise conveys a wealth of benefits, many of them psychological as well as physical. A must for everyone, exercise is particularly important to those who suffer from chronic, potentially debilitating diseases such as arthritis.

What are some of the specific benefits of regular exercise?

Working out on a regular basis is helpful in many, many ways. Regular exercise:

- Slows the debilitating process of arthritis

- Strengthens the muscles and other structures around your joints, providing greater stability

- Keeps your joints moving

- Enhances cartilage and bone strength

- Reduces pain

- Helps you maintain an ideal body weight

- Increases your range of motion

- Enables you to accomplish daily activities with greater energy, strength, and flexibility

- Helps you sleep better

- Releases feel-good chemicals called endorphins in your brain

- Boosts your energy level

- Increases your sense of well-being

- Builds your self-confidence

- Helps control stress, anxiety, and depression

What's the best way to get started?

Especially if you've been inactive, it's best to start out slowly. Before you put on your walking shoes, be sure to consult your physician. Only your doctor can tell you what's safe for you and what's not.

I've heard that exercise can be dangerous when you have arthritis. Is this true?

Not if you go about it in the right way. But some of us make mistakes such as trying to jump-start an exercise program by doing too much too soon. This is unwise, for it may result in further joint damage and pain.

Are there any other pitfalls to avoid?

Yes. Don't let yourself fall into the weekend warrior trap. Some of us sit at our desks all week and then try to make up for it by going all out on Saturday or Sunday. This is a mistake that can lead to further joint damage, aches, pains, strains, and sprains. But don't get discouraged. If you begin an exercise program carefully and responsibly and stick with it on a regular basis, the odds are that you'll meet with success.

What should I do if I experience pain as a result of exercise?

If you ever feel dizzy, short of breath, or experience chest pain, stop exercising at once and consult your doctor. These can be the warning signs of a heart attack.

What if exercise leads to more joint pain and swelling?

Take a break. Gently massage sore muscles to loosen painful cramps, or apply an ice pack to ease inflammation. Medication such as analgesics, nonselective NSAIDs, and COX-2 inhibitors can also help see you through difficult patches. In this chapter you'll learn a variety of self-help strategies—such as warming up, pacing yourself, and using heat and cold—to prevent injuries during exercise. Of course, whenever the pain is severe or if these measures don't help, stop exercising—at least for now—and see your doctor.

I have a full-time job and two children. How can I possibly fit in the time to exercise?

People have many reasons for not exercising. Beyond family and career, you may be too tired, it may be raining out, or you may not belong to a gym. Your joints may feel too achy and sore, or maybe you just don't like to exercise. You're far from alone in your reluctance, for we live in a country full of couch potatoes. But some form of exercise is vital to everyone, especially those who have arthritis. Make it a priority to fit exercise into your daily routine. Set the alarm clock for half an hour earlier and begin your day with gentle stretches. Spend your lunch hour at the gym swimming laps instead of munching on a ham and cheese sandwich, or at the end of the day fit in a walk around the neighborhood with your spouse.

Can incorporating more movement into my daily lifestyle replace regular exercise?

Unfortunately, no. When you have arthritis, you need to participate in a number of different kinds of exercises. Taking the stairs instead of the elevator, walking to the corner store instead of driving, and doing housework all burn calories and can help you keep extra pounds off—but they will not help you maintain your flexibility. As you'll learn, only range-of-motion (ROM) exercises can help you accomplish this.

BALANCE EXERCISE WITH REST

What happens when my arthritis flares up?

During a flare, affected joints become warm, painful, and swollen. When this happens, you must get some rest to reduce inflammation. Don't be bashful about asking for help from your friends and family. Whenever you feel the need, take a guilt-free afternoon nap. During these periods, you may feel more comfortable wearing a supportive splint.

Should I stop exercising altogether during flares?

When in doubt, ask your doctor. But even during most flares, you can still perform very gentle range-of-motion exercises to maintain joint movement. Depending on how you feel, you may also want to add isometric exercises for muscle strength.

I have severe rheumatoid arthritis. How can I tell what balance of exercise, activity, and rest is right for me?

Only your health-care team can help you strike the right balance of therapeutic exercise, activity, and rest. Therapeutic exercises are essential to keep your joints flexible, your muscles strong, and your heart and lungs fit. But these must be balanced with an ability to meet your normal obligations: the day-to-day activities involved in your job, family and child-care needs, and leisure time. And rest is essential, especially during flares.

EXERCISE AND OSTEOPOROSIS

I'm in my fifties and worried about developing osteoporosis. Can weight-bearing exercise help prevent this?

Yes. Although it's best to start weight-bearing exercise at an early age and make it part of your lifetime exercise program, it's never too late to get started (after getting the okay from your doctor, of course). Weight-bearing exercise helps build bone, which can slow down or halt the progression of this dangerous, bone-thinning disease.

What are some examples of weight-bearing exercise?

Any exercises that have an impact on bones are helpful. For example, walking and dancing are good weight-bearing exercises. With the approval of your doctor or therapist, carry a 1-pound weight in each hand to improve your walking workouts. Swimming, healthy as it is in so many other ways, is not a very good weight-bearing exercise. If your arthritis feels better when you work out in a heated pool, join a warm-water exercise program. (Contact your local Arthritis Foundation branch to see where classes are available in your area.)

I have lupus. Should I be particularly concerned about osteoporosis?

Yes. Women who have inflammatory rheumatoid arthritis or lupus are especially prone to developing osteoporosis, because of the nature of the diseases themselves and because they are often treated with corticosteroids. Long-term treatment with corticosteroids is known to lead to brittle bones.

Is it really necessary to see my doctor before starting a new exercise program?

Yes. It's absolutely essential to consult with your doctor before beginning any new workout. Although even people who have severe arthritis or osteoporosis can benefit from some form of exercise, only your doctor can determine the levels of movement and exertion that are best for you. You'll need to learn what kinds of exercises are beneficial, and those that may prove dangerous to your condition.

YOUR HEALTH-CARE TEAM

How will my doctor determine what type of exercise program is right for me?

This depends on the type of arthritis you have, which joints are affected, and your degree of disability.

What other medical professionals might participate in these decisions?

In many cases, your doctor acts as the head of a cooperative health-care team. Following a careful physical examination, he may refer you to another team member for further evaluation, information, and treatment. In close consultation with your doctor, a specialist such as a physiatrist, physical therapist, or occupational therapist can design an individualized exercise program for you. These specialists can teach you what exercises are beneficial to you and alert you to those that can end up doing more harm than good.

How can a physiatrist help me?

A physiatrist is a medical doctor who specializes in physical rehabilitation. Especially when your arthritis has resulted in severe disability, a physiatrist can design a comprehensive rehabilitation program for you. This may consist of techniques such as physical therapy, regular exercise, hot and cold packs, and transcutaneous electrical nerve stimulation (TENS) to relieve pain. Because physiatrists are medical doctors, they can prescribe drugs as necessary. They also emphasize education about arthritis and proper body mechanics.

What can an occupational therapist do for me?

Occupational therapists are trained in ergonomics, or body mechanics: the science of moving your body in the proper way. They can teach you how to sit, stand, lift, and move around without placing undue stress and strain on your joints. When necessary, occupational therapists can fit you with splints, braces, and other supportive devices designed to protect your joints during therapeutic exercise or day-to-day activity.

How can a physical therapist help me?

Physical therapists are medical professionals who can show you how to correctly perform the exercises that, over time, will give you greater strength in your muscles and bones and increased flexibility in your joints. A good exercise program can relieve your present pain and help prevent future flares from occurring. Physical therapists also use a variety of other techniques to help you feel better.

What other kinds of techniques do physical therapists use?

Treatments such as heat and ice massage, regular massage, hydrotherapy, transcutaneous electrical nerve stimulation (TENS), and ultrasound increase the flow of blood and oxygen to painful muscles and joints, generating heat and offering soothing pain relief.

What is TENS?

Transcutaneous electrical nerve stimulation, or TENS, is a therapy in which electrodes attached to the skin transmit a painless, low-voltage current. As a result, you feel a kind of tingling sensation. In stimulating nerves, the current is believed to distract the brain from noticing pain.

Who usually administers TENS treatments?

TENS treatments may be given by physiatrists, physical therapists, or occupational therapists. A therapist can also train you to use a TENS unit at home.

What is the difference between regular exercise and physical therapy?

- Regular exercise consists of stretching or swimming or walking or going to an aerobics class. Although your doctor or therapist may advise you how to best go about regular exercise, this is not physical therapy.

- Physical therapy takes place when you injure yourself, experience severe swelling and joint pain, or following surgery. The therapist performs ankle, knee, hip, shoulder, elbow, or wrist movements with you, depending on the nature of your problem. In each case, a special program of physical therapy is carefully tailored to fit the individual's needs.

What about physical therapy in the water? Is that good for my arthritis?

Yes it is. Strengthening exercises in the water promote active movement across a joint without putting a lot of stress on it.

How does physical therapy in the water work?

Most aquatic therapy sessions begin and end with several minutes of water-walking to allow you to warm up and cool down. During therapy, gentle bending and stretching movements are performed as you either stand up or float (supported by your therapist and using flotation devices), according to techniques called vertical stabilization and Bad Ragaz. In a relatively short time, aquatic therapy can lead to reduced swelling and a greater range of movement in target joints.

How are physical and occupational therapists different from doctors? And how are they different from one another?

Therapists are often affiliated with hospital rehabilitation centers, but they are not doctors and cannot prescribe drugs. In some cases, you will find that the roles of physical and occupational therapists overlap. In general, occupational therpists teach you how to put as little stress as possible on your joints as you go about your day-to-day activities. Physical therapists perform movements with you and teach you special exercise techniques to keep your joints flexible and your muscles strong.

ANTI-ARTHRITIS EXERCISES

What types of exercise are most helpful in coping with arthritis?

Three different forms of exercise are most useful:

- **Range-of-motion (ROM) exercises** reduce stiffness and keep joints flexible.

- **Strengthening exercises** increase the strength of muscles and other tissues that stabilize joints.

- **Aerobic or endurance exercise** builds overall fitness.

I haven't exercised in years. After my doctor gives me the go-ahead, what are the best exercises to begin with?

If you're out of shape or if you are experiencing pain and stiffness, start with range-of-motion and strengthening exercises. Once you feel comfortable with these movements, which are the easiest on your body, begin incorporating small amounts of aerobic activity into your workouts.

How often should I exercise?

The Arthritis Foundation recommends that you do your range-of-motion exercises every day, and your strengthening and aerobic exercises every other day.

RANGE-OF-MOTION EXERCISES

What are range-of-motion exercises?

These are stretching exercises designed to keep the highest possible degree of flexibility in your joints. Your range of motion is the full extent to which any joint can normally move in different directions. ROM exercises help you maintain and potentially increase the range of motion of your joints.

How are range-of-motion exercises helpful?

By stretching the tissue around affected joints, ROM exercises help prevent the muscles, ligaments, and tendons from bending, tightening, and locking your joints into deformed positions. Repetitions help to relieve stiffness, maintain flexibility, and keep movement pain-free.

What types of ROM exercises are helpful?

There are a number of different ROM exercises, each designed to open up and stretch different parts

of the body. Your health-care team will determine
which are best for you.

What are some examples of ROM exercises?

To benefit your knees and hips, lie on your back
and draw alternate knees to your chest. To enhance
finger flexibility, touch each finger to the tip of your
thumb to form complete circles.

How vigorously should I perform ROM exercises?

Your movements should be as gentle and fluid as
possible. Don't force anything. If you bounce or move
beyond comfort while performing range-of-motion
exercises, you risk harming your joints.

STRENGTHENING EXERCISE

What are strengthening exercises? How can they help manage arthritis?

A well-designed, regular program of strengthening
exercises can help you maintain or even increase muscle strength. Strength is the amount of force a muscle
puts forth. When you have arthritis, strong muscles
are especially important to stabilize your joints. Ne-
glected muscles can weaken, leaving you open to all
sorts of injury. Isometric, isotonic, and isokinetic are
three helpful strengthening exercises.

What are isometric exercises?

In performing isometric exercises, you tighten your muscles and then relax them without moving your joints. These exercises promote stability and are a good choice when your joints are swollen and inflamed.

What are isotonic exercises?

When you do isotonic exercises, you move your joints in order to strengthen your muscles. Although they resemble ROM exercises, isotonic exercises add both strength and flexibility because the repetitions are performed more quickly. When you are ready, and subject to the approval of your doctor or therapist, add light 1- or 2-pound weights to your workouts. To minimize stress to joints and take advantage of its natural resistance, some people like to do isotonic exercise in the water.

What are isokinetic exercises?

These are essentially isotonic exercises performed on exercise or weight machines. Available at most gyms, you can add or subtract weights from machines to achieve the desired level of resistance. Low weights at high speeds increase your endurance, while heavier weights at slower speeds increase your strength.

AEROBIC EXERCISE

What is aerobic exercise?

Aerobic or endurance exercise builds overall fitness. Regular walking, swimming, or bicycling increases the flow of oxygen through your body, strengthening the heart and lungs, and is very helpful in controlling arthritis. Aerobic exercises can help you manage pain, improve joint function, increase stamina, and strengthen your muscles to give your joints greater stability.

I get sore and out of breath very quickly doing aerobic exercises. How often do I really have to do them? And for how long?

First, choose an aerobic activity that you like to do. If you're enjoying yourself, you're less likely to feel these discomforts. Begin with just five minutes of aerobic exercise each day. Then gradually work your way up to three five-minute periods of exercise, for a grand total of 15 minutes. Over time, make it your goal to extend workouts to 30 minutes at a time every other day.

I walk on a regular basis, and I'm trying to step up my routine. How will I know if I'm overdoing it?

Take the "talk test." To get the most out of your walk it's important to set the right pace. A good rule of thumb is that you should be able to talk while you walk. If you're panting or gasping or you can't catch your breath to chat with a buddy at the top of a hill, you're working too hard. Slow down and give your heart and lungs a chance to work up to more intense walks and climbs.

Can aerobic exercise help me control my weight?

Yes. Walking, swimming, or bicycling several times a week can help you keep those extra pounds from accumulating as you grow older.

What does being overweight have to do with arthritis?

Being overweight increases your risk of developing arthritis, and it aggravates arthritis if you already have it. Osteoarthritis arises about twice as often among people who are obese (that is, who weigh 20% more than their ideal weight) than among those of normal weight. When you're overweight, you also face a greater risk of developing gout.

I suffer from osteoarthritis, and must admit I'm a few pounds overweight. Should I go on a diet?

Extra pounds mean extra pressure and stress on weight-bearing joints such as hips and knees, which can accelerate damage to cartilage. This means that you should try to lose a few pounds, but it does not mean that you should go on any crazy diets. The sensible route to lasting weight loss is cutting back on calories and saturated fats and getting regular exercise.

What are the best kinds of aerobic exercise for people who have arthritis?

Walking, aquatic aerobics, and riding on a stationary bicycle are three excellent exercises. They are easy on your joints as well as beneficial to your overall fitness.

Are there any types of exercises that I should avoid?

Depending on your particular physical limitations, some activities may become off-limits to you. For instance, running has a high impact on the weight-bearing joints. Although many people who have arthritis continue to jog, walking is a considerably safer alternative. Tennis is stressful to shoulder and elbow joints, while the twisting movements of golf are hard on the spine.

I love tennis and can't stand the thought of giving it up. What should I do?

Talk to your doctor or physical therapist. Sometimes the physical and psychological benefits of participating in sports you enjoy outweigh their risk.

AQUATIC EXERCISE

What is aquatic exercise?

Aquatic exercise, or performing exercises in the water, is one of the best workout alternatives for people with arthritis. The soothing properties of water combine to make it especially easy on aching joints, and the heated pool at your local health club or YMCA may be just the place for you to get moving again.

What types of aquatic exercise are available?

There are a number of different ways of working out in the water. They include:

• Aquatic therapy with a physical therapist

• Swimming

• Water walking

• Aquatic aerobics class

What makes water such a happy medium for people who have arthritis?

Water does not place stress on your weight-bearing joints. Its effects are soothing and healing, in sharp contrast to the jarring impact of many land-based activities.

How are the physical properties of water beneficial to arthritis sufferers?

The buoyancy, resistance, pressure, and warmth of water unite to create a therapeutic environment uniquely well-suited to physical healing and emotional relaxation.

How is the buoyancy of water helpful?

Because buoyancy exerts a force opposite to gravity, you actually weigh less in water than on land. Buoyancy allows water to act like a giant cushion—surrounding, protecting, and reducing stress on your aching joints. By taking the pressure off joints, buoyancy enables you to exercise through a greater range of motion.

What does water's resistance add to its healing qualities?

A very important element of buoyancy is resistance, which can help you build muscle strength and tone. As you swim, walk, or perform exercises in the water, you can feel yourself moving against the gentle but persistent resistance of water. In addition to strengthening your muscles, moving your limbs against the water gives you a good cardiovascular workout and can keep your weight down.

Why is it safer to perform my strengthening exercises in the water?

Strengthening exercises in the water promote active movement across a joint without putting a lot of stress on it. In this way, water's gentle resistance protects you from the worrisome injuries associated with high-impact exercises performed on land.

How is water pressure helpful to sore and swollen joints?

Water exerts pressure in all directions, with a soothing effect on your muscles that is much like a therapeutic massage. The pressure of water helps reduce painful swelling and inflammation, strengthens joints, and improves circulation in your extremities. When there is swelling in the soft tissue around a joint, immersing it in water is like wrapping it in a giant bandage.

What role does water temperature play?

Warm water increases the blood flow in joints and relieves muscle pain. As you relax in warm water, your breathing becomes more rhythmic, and your muscles and joints slowly grow more supple and limber. Warm water between 83 and 90 degrees is ideal for decreasing pain and promoting relaxation.

What are the health benefits of swimming?

Moving your limbs against the resistance of the water strengthens your heart and lungs, while buoyancy safely cushions your joints. Swimming works all the major muscle groups, firming and toning the body, lowering stress and blood pressure, and increasing the level of your "good" HDL cholesterol.

What about aqua aerobics?

Aqua aerobics—aerobics classes in the pool—offer the same health benefits as classes in the gym without the accompanying risk of impact injuries. A water aerobics program can help you increase flexibility and range of motion in your joints, while enhancing your overall strength and cardiovascular fitness. Freedom of movement in the water makes possible a greater range of motion. Of course, be careful not to get carried away and overdo.

How about water-walking?

Many YMCAs, health clubs, and community fitness centers across the country set aside designated hours and outer lanes of pools for water walkers. Some even place a hand rail at waist level for added support. If you don't like to swim or just feel like a change, walking in chest-deep water supports most of your body weight and can provide the same joint-strengthening effects.

How can I find out what warm-water exercise activities are available in my area?

Call your local branch of the Arthritis Foundation.

STRATEGIES FOR SAFE EXERCISE

Are there any special safety tips I should follow when exercising?

Try these helpful strategies:

- Warm up and cool down with range-of-motion and strengthening exercises.

- Wear loose, comfortable clothing and well-fitting shoes.

- Breathe in and breathe out when you exercise. Don't hold your breath.

- Stop exercising if you experience shortness of breath, dizziness, or chest pain.

- Don't try to do too much too soon.

- Use heat or cold (or alternate them) over muscles and joints to provide short-term relief from pain and stiffness.

HEAT AND COLD TREATMENTS

What makes heat and cold especially helpful when it comes to arthritis?

Heat relieves stiffness and pain, while cold reduces pain and swelling.

When are heat and cold helpful?

Heat and cold treatments can be helpful both before and after exercising.

Are there any special precautions I should follow?

Heat treatments should be comfortably warm, but not too hot. Ice should never be applied directly to the skin. Wrap it in a towel first to prevent frostbite.

How is ice useful?

The immediate application of an ice pack after an injury will provide much-needed relief of the often intense initial pain. In addition, ice will reduce internal bleeding and swelling by decreasing blood flow. If you don't have an ice pack, just put a few ice cubes in a plastic bag or use a package of frozen vegetables. If you have recurrent arthritis pain, try keeping a reusable commercial cold pack from your local drugstore in the freezer.

How can I safely use ice treatments?

Be careful not to leave ice on the skin for too long. If your skin grows numb, it's time to remove the ice, at least temporarily, to avoid frostbite.

How is heat helpful?

Hot, moist compresses or towels, commercial hot packs, hot water bottles, heating pads, heat lamps, and hot baths and showers can all act as effective heat applications. For acute back pain, alternate them with ice therapy. You can also try visiting your gym for some gentle stretches and a swim in the heated pool, and then top off your back-friendly workout with a relaxing break in the steam room or hot tub.

What are some helpful ways to use heat and cold?

Try these strategies:

- Take a warm shower or bath shortly before your workout to relax your joints and muscles and ease inflammation.

- Apply a warm compress, hot pack, heating pad, or heat lamp to sore joints.

- Sit in a warm whirlpool.

- Wrap a cold pack, bag of ice, or bag of frozen vegetables in a towel and place it on achy joints.

STAYING MOTIVATED

I get frustrated just thinking about all the exercises I'm supposed to do. What should I focus on to start with?

Frequency and consistency are the most important elements when you're getting started. Even if it's only for a short time, make yourself put on your walking shoes, open the front door, and take a walk around the block. Make a workout schedule, and stick to it. Later on there will be plenty of time to concentrate on your form and add more intensity to your workout.

I'm so out of shape and my joints are weak and sore. Is it still possible for me to begin an exercise program?

Most likely yes, but be sure to see your doctor first. When joints are sore or weakened, it's best to start extra slowly and carefully. Aquatic exercise, so easy on the joints, may be a good place for you to begin. If you opt for walking instead, be sure to invest in proper equipment such as high-topped shoes to support your ankles. Ask your doctor or therapist about wearing over-the-counter elastic supports or sleeve braces to protect your joints.

I have great intentions, but no matter how hard I try I get bored with my workouts. How do I stay motivated and maintain my exercise program?

Over time it can be a real challenge to keep up with regular exercise, so try strategies like these to keep interested and stay motivated:

- **Set short-term and long-term goals.** Measure how many laps you swim or miles you walk and keep track of them in a fitness journal. If you're not sure how much ground you cover walking, calculate your mileage by checking the distance on your car's odometer. Alternatively, invest in a small, portable odometer and attach it to your belt. Clocking how many miles you go can be very satisfying. As you reach each goal outlined in your journal, reward yourself with a special trip to your favorite restaurant or a night out at the movies.

• **Buddy up.** Going to the gym or water-walking and talking with a good friend can give your spirits as well as your body a welcome boost. You're also more likely to keep on a regular exercise schedule if someone else is counting on you to be there.

• **Be prepared.** Schedule your exercise at a consistent time and lay out your swimsuit or sneakers in advance. Many experts advise working out in the mornings to make sure that you fit exercise into your busy schedule. If your joints are up to it, a morning workout can also give you an extra burst of energy to start your day.

• **Buy a heart-rate monitor.** A monitor can help you determine when you reach the heart-rate zone that is most optimal to your health. If you're not fond of gadgets but would still like to work toward a training level, learn how to take your heart rate at the local gym.

• **Invest in a portable cassette or CD player.** If you hit the road on your own, listening to music or books on tape is a good way to keep moving.

Of course, always make sure that you watch out for traffic when you do this.

- **Vary your routine.** If you're a biker, choose different routes through your park or neighborhood. If you prefer walking, on a weekend day take a more ambitious hike in the mountains or a sunrise walk on the beach. If you're hooked on the heated pool at your club, you can still mix it up. Do a water aerobics class one day, and for your next workout walk or swim laps.

NINE

❖❖❖

Managing Your Day-To-Day Activities

When you have arthritis, your mental and physical well-being both suffer. But I've taught myself to keep looking for answers. For example, when my arthritis prevented me from getting out to the library, I got an Internet connection. And when I saw an ad about participating in clinical trials for a new arthritis medication, I answered it.

Laurie Schuster, 37-year-old osteoarthritis patient
and participant in Celebrex clinical trials

The pain and inflammation of arthritis can make it difficult to manage even the most basic day-to-day activities. You may have trouble getting out of bed in the morning or buttoning your shirt. Swollen fingers may thwart your ability to perform such basic actions as picking up the phonebook and dialing a number. Negotiating a flight of stairs, cooking a meal, or pruning a bush in your garden may seem like daunting tasks. The growing debilitation of arthritis can eventually rob you of your independence—but you don't have to allow that to happen. In this chapter, you'll learn about many basic self-care skills to protect your joints.

PROTECT YOUR JOINTS

How can I avoid placing excess stress on my joints?

The Arthritis Foundation recommends these three general methods of joint protection:

- **Pay attention to joint position.** This means using strongest joints and larger muscle groups to lift things.

- **Plan ahead.** Organize your day and manage your time efficiently.

- **Pace yourself.** Alternate periods of activity with periods of rest.

Because my joints ache, my instinct is to keep them still. Do I really have to move them?

A proper balance of rest, day-to-day activity, and exercise is best. When you are experiencing a painful flare, your instinct is correct: Don't put extra pressure on joints that are already inflamed. But protecting your joints does not mean neglecting to move them altogether. On the contrary, over time this will make joints stiffen up even more and cause the muscles around them to weaken. The trick is to learn how to move your joints sensibly and responsibly. Your doctor, occupational therapist, or other member of your health-care team is the best person to teach you valuable joint-sparing techniques.

How do I know when it is best to rest and when I should move around?

Try to tune in to the needs of your own body. Listen to its signals. When your body tells you that you are hungry, you eat. Likewise, when your body tells you that you are tired and your swollen joints ache, you should allow yourself time to rest and heal.

What should I do if I'm in pain?

Pain is your body's signal to you that something is wrong. If day-to-day activities or exercise aggravate your pain, slow down. You probably got carried away and did too much. Do a little less next time, and if you continue to experience pain see your physician.

What is a good balance of activity and rest?

The proper balance of rest, activity, and exercise naturally varies from person to person, and so it is best decided with the aid of your health-care team.

What's the difference between normal activity and exercise?

Your day-to-day activities begin with getting out of bed and getting dressed every day—no easy task when you suffer from morning stiffness. Your many other activities might include preparing meals, working at your job, caring for your family, doing household chores, or driving your car. As you'll learn in this chapter, there are special joint-sparing strategies that you can employ in all these cases. But also keep in mind that day-to-day activities are not a replacement for the stretching, strengthening, and aerobic exercises that you should perform on a regular basis to help manage your arthritis.

Why do my joints stiffen up?

It may be helpful to think of your body like a machine—for example, a car. You need to put oil in your car and run the engine on a regular basis, for cars grow rusty from disuse. An engine with little oil runs roughly. If you force your vehicle to run without oil, you will burn out the engine.

Likewise, you need to take good care of your body. The way to keep the joints in your body healthy and well lubricated is with regular movement. When you use them on a regular basis, joints will function more efficiently and give you less pain. When you don't move them for a long period of time, joints grow creaky, stiff, and tired. They may even freeze. Muscles hurt as well after doing activity or exercise that you aren't used to. The more inactive you are, the greater your risk of injury in carrying out your regular daily activities.

Is good posture important too?

Yes. Good posture protects your joints, while bad posture is tiring and adds to pain. Unfortunately, many people mistakenly believe that good posture consists of standing at attention. Not so. Shoulders should not be jammed all the way back. Instead, relax your arms. Stack your shoulders, hips, knees, and heels in one imaginary straight column. Tuck in your buttocks and lift your ribcage. (This has the added benefit of making you look thinner.) Pull your belly button in and unround your shoulders. Avoid the temptation to lock your knees. Place your feet hip-width apart, with toes pointing forward.

Standing for long periods of time makes my arthritis act up. What can I do to avoid this?

Put a foot up. This takes the pressure off your joints and keeps you from slouching. Keep a short stool handy to rest your foot on, or lean against a wall.

Is sitting for long periods tough on the joints?

It can be. "If I sit at my computer for an hour straight, I'm stiff when I get up," says osteoarthritis sufferer and Celebrex patient Laurie Stollery. "I feel much better when I take regular breaks and walk around for a few minutes." Like Laurie, try to break up periods of extended sitting or standing with short walks. This takes the pressure off stiff and achy joints.

If your knees bother you, Laurie also recommends putting your feet up when you watch TV.

After taking a COX-2 inhibitor for several months, my arthritis is no longer bothering me. Is it okay to stop taking my medication?

No. Your arthritis is most likely under control because you are regularly taking a COX-2 inhibitor or other arthritis medication. To stop would probably mean a return of painful symptoms.

Should I take additional COX-2 inhibitors when my arthritis is acting up?

No. Take COX-2 inhibitors or other arthritis medications exactly as prescribed or recommended by your physician.

What other strategies can help me successfully manage my day-to-day activities?

Reaching out to friends and family for help is essential. There are also many self-help strategies you can employ to protect your joints.

ASK FAMILY AND FRIENDS FOR HELP

What role can my friends and family play in helping me cope with arthritis?

It's vital to share your needs, concerns, and feelings about arthritis with your family and close friends.

Don't shut them out of what you are going through. In many cases, they may be even more worried and confused than you are.

Are support groups helpful?

In many cases, yes. It's often very comforting to know that you are not alone. In the company of others who suffer from the same problems and concerns as you do, you can share your experiences and exchange tips on how to best go about coping with the challenges of arthritis.

Are there any courses available to help me learn more about managing my arthritis?

In many areas around the country, the Arthritis Foundation offers self-help classes to help you take control of your own care. The Arthritis Foundation has over 150 local offices. Phone (800) 283-7800 to locate the office nearest you, and give them a call.

IN THE OFFICE

Is it important to design a safe and comfortable work area?

It's essential to do this in order to prevent sore shoulders, an aching back, and painful wrists.

- Sit in an adjustable chair with comfortable armrests.

- Place a lumbar pillow or rolled-up towel behind your back for support.

- If your feet don't reach the floor when you sit at your desk, use a footstool or box.

- To keep your muscles relaxed, shift your weight occasionally.

- Get up to walk around and stretch every half hour or so.

- Keep your computer monitor at eye level. You should be able to look down at the screen rather than up at it, which strains your eyes and neck.

- Place the computer keyboard so that your arms are at 90 degrees to the body. Install wrist rests.

- Keep the mouse close at hand—reaching puts stress on arms and shoulders.

- Keep files and supplies within easy reach.

- Use reaching devices instead of bending or stretching to grasp hard-to-reach objects.

- Use felt-tipped and large-barrel pens.

- If you use the phone a lot, get a headset.

AROUND THE HOUSE

What techniques can I use around the house to ease excess pressure on my joints?

Try these strategies:

- If you have arthritis in your knees or back, use chairs with armrests. When you get up, hoist yourself up with your arms rather than putting pressure on your knees and spine.

- Choose long-handled vacuums, mops, and other household helpers. Extensions are also helpful in avoiding painful stooping and reaching.

- Dust and wash with mitts.

- Wear comfortable shoes with low heels. Tight shoes and high heels can aggravate arthritic pain.

- Organize your home so that what you need is within easy reach.

- Store cleaning supplies on a cart.

- When possible, sit on a stool to perform chores such as washing dishes or ironing clothes.

Is it important to use the right body mechanics?

Yes. There are a number of ways to do this:

- Hold items that you are lifting close to your body.

- Learn to lift objects the right way. Keeping your back straight, bend your knees, and lift by straightening up your legs.

- Avoid any unnecessary bending and twisting. When possible, push or slide items such as furniture across the floor instead of trying to lift and carry them.

- Keep moving. Change positions frequently to prevent stiffness.

I have rheumatoid arthritis and have terrible trouble with my fingers. What can I do to make my life easier?

Try these finger-saving tips recommended by the Arthritis Foundation:

- Avoid any activities that require a tight grip.

- Try not to put too much direct pressure on your fingers.

- Steer clear of pinching, squeezing, and twisting motions.

IN THE KITCHEN

What special anti-arthritis strategies can I use in the kitchen?

Because we spend so much time in the kitchen, it's essential to get organized and arrange your drawers and cupboards as efficiently as possible. Also try to plan your weekly meals so that you have everything on hand and don't have to make unnecessary trips out to the grocery store.

Try these helpful strategies:

- Organize your closet shelves so that the most frequently used items are within easy reach. Store heavy items at waist level.

- Install pull-out shelves to gain even easier access to closet space.

- Place magnetic hooks on the refrigerator and hang pot holders from them.

- If cabinet doors are hard to open, remove magnetic catches from them. Install easy-to-grasp knobs or handles on the outsides of closets and cupboards.

- Wear an apron with deep pockets to keep the supplies you need close at hand.

- To get the top off that stubborn jar of peanut butter, rest it on a rubber pad. Use rubber gloves to help get a good grip on lids.

- Make liberal use of appliances such as dishwashers, microwaves, can openers, food processors, and mixers to give your joints a break.

- If you have trouble gripping dishes with your fingers, wear oven mitts.

- Invest in utensils with wide handles that you can wrap your fingers around.

- If you have trouble holding a glass, use a straw.

- When you carry a bag of groceries, use your arms instead of your fingers to avoid putting excess strain on their joints.

- Choose lightweight, nonstick pots and pans. Use types such as Pyrex that you can cook in, serve from, and deposit directly in the dishwasher.

- For easier cleanup, use disposable aluminum roasting pans, cookie sheets, and baking dishes.

- Use a long-necked spatula or tongs to turn food in the oven.

- Put a foot up. Standing with both feet flat is hard on your back. If you have to stand for long periods while cooking or washing the dishes, rest one foot on a low stool. Better yet, whenever possible sit on a stool while cooking or washing.

- Plan your meals in advance. In addition to saving yourself extra trips, you can devise a more nutritious menu for yourself and your family. While this is a good idea for everyone, it's especially important for arthritis sufferers. As you probably know all too well, pain, fatigue, and lack of appetite can lead to poor nutrition.

- Double your recipes and freeze the leftovers.

IN THE BATHROOM

I'm worried about slipping and hurting myself in the bathroom. How can I keep this from happening?

There are many ways to protect yourself from injury in the bathroom. Try the following:

- Install handrails in the tub and beside the toilet.

- Use lever-type faucets.

- Place rubber mats inside and outside the bathtub, and consider investing in a small plastic stool or a transfer bench so you can sit while showering.

- Buy an electric toothbrush with a built-up handle. Less rigorous movement is required than with normal toothbrushes and their handles are thicker and easier to grip. If an electric toothbrush is too heavy, wrap a piece of padding around the handle of your regular toothbrush.

- If it's difficult to get toothpaste from the tube, lean on it or squeeze it between your palms.

- Keep your soap, shampoo, and conditioner centrally organized in a shower caddy.

- Add a detachable showerhead for easier rinsing and maybe even the occasional massage.

IN THE BEDROOM

Is getting a good night's sleep helpful?

Absolutely. Getting restorative sleep is essential for everyone who has arthritis, especially those who suffer from fibromyalgia. A number of natural strategies can help you sleep more contentedly:

- Be sure you have a comfortable bed and a supportive pillow.

- Keep your bedroom completely dark and as free of noise as possible. Use a white noise generator, a water fountain, or tapes of nature sounds such as ocean or rain to block out noise.

- Choose lightweight quilts to keep heavy, uncomfortable covers off your feet.

- If you sleep on your back, alleviate potential discomforts by placing pillows under your knees. Likewise, place a pillow under your upper leg if you sleep on your side.

- Go to bed at night and get up in the morning at the same times, even on weekends, to help your body establish a normal rhythm.

- Don't drink coffee or alcohol in the evening.

- In the hour before you go to sleep, avoid stimulants such as the TV, computer, and bright lights.

- Take a warm bath just before retiring.

- Set aside an hour before bedtime to read quietly to yourself.

- Don't bring reading material from work into bed with you.

- Reserve the news for daytime or early evening review. Don't watch evening newscasts or read newspapers right before trying to go to sleep.

- Don't take sleeping pills unless your physician recommends or prescribes them.

- Do see your doctor if in spite of all your efforts you cannot get a good night's sleep.

What about getting dressed?

- Wear loose-fitting clothing.

- Sit down when you get dressed.

- Use a long-handled shoehorn.

- Buy sneakers with Velcro fasteners instead of shoelaces.

- Attach large paper clips to zippers to make them easier to fasten and unfasten.

Are there any helpful tips for dealing with sexual problems associated with arthritis?

If sexual activity is affected by your arthritis, try to share your concerns about this. Be open and honest with your partner. When necessary, ask your doctor to provide specific suggestions to help you cope with your problems.

IN THE GARDEN

Soothing as gardening may be to the psyche, it is hard on the knees. Try these joint-saving strategies:

- Use a kneeling pad to cushion your knees or sit on a small stool to reduce bending. Combination kneeler/seats and lightweight benches with side grips are available from gardening catalogs.

- Use ergonomic hand tools with rotating handles. These special tools rotate on an axis to follow the motion of your hand. In so doing, they reduce the amount your wrist must flex as you hold the tool.

- Invest in long handles. When shopping for a rake, avoid stooping and reaching by choosing one with a long handle or extension.

ON THE ROAD

Long drives are notoriously hard on the back. When you're on the road, make it easier on your joints by using tips like these:

- Opt for power steering, windows, and seats in your car.

- Invest in an automatic garage opener.

- If turning keys is a problem, build up their tops or use key holders. A lever-type car door opener is another alternative.

- On long drives, slip a lumbar pillow or a rolled-up towel behind your lower back. The extra support will prevent or ease low back pain. Also consider a horseshoe-shaped pillow to cushion and protect your neck and head.

- When you have difficulty turning your neck, use a wide-angled mirror.

WHEN YOU TRAVEL

Are there any special precautions that I should take when I travel?

Arthritis need not deter you from taking a business or pleasure trip. There are some very simple steps you can take to prevent your arthritis from flaring up while you're on the move:

- Pack lightly. Do yourself a favor by keeping the weight of your suitcase to a minimum, and invest in luggage on wheels to further ease your burden. If you have to carry a bag, drape the shoulder straps across your body to evenly distribute its weight and keep your hands free.

- When making plane reservations, ask for a bulk-head seat. These have substantially more leg room. In flight, avoid stiffness by periodically getting up and walking around.

- On planes or trains, as in cars, place a lumbar pillow or a rolled-up towel behind your lower back for extra support. This can help prevent or relieve arthritis pain, especially low back pain. A horseshoe-shaped pillow can help cushion and protect your neck and head.

- Choose an arthritis-friendly hotel. Amenities such as heated pools and whirlpools can go a long way toward helping you enjoy that business trip or vacation.

TEN
🔷🔷🔷🔷

Alternative Treatments for Arthritis

Before I started taking Celebrex, I tried some alternatives. I wore copper around my wrist for a while, but it didn't really help any.

Frank Edwards, 57-year-old osteoarthritis and
rheumatoid arthritis patient and participant
in Celebrex clinical trials

While most people who have arthritis benefit from medications like COX-2 inhibitors and strategies such as pain and stress management, joint protection, and regular exercise, rarely do symptoms completely disappear. This leads many arthritis sufferers to seek out alternative remedies to soothe chronic pain and inflammation, to enhance immune function, or to get a much-needed good night's sleep.

THE ALTERNATIVES

Aside from standard approaches like medication and exercise, what other treatments are available to help people who have arthritis?

Alternatives run the gamut from the sensible to the outlandish. They include the very popular dietary supplements glucosamine and chondroitin as well as stress-management techniques like meditation, visualization, and guided imagery. All of these have been demonstrated to be of some help to at least some arthritis sufferers.

And then there are the more offbeat alternatives, such as wearing copper bracelets or ingesting bee and ant venom. Over the years, as one of the oldest known and most painful chronic illnesses, arthritis has inspired folk remedies including daily bee stings, tablespoons of cod liver or snake oil, or eating nine gin-soaked raisins a day. Some people still swear by their gin-soaked raisins.

How can I tell whether it is safe to try an alternative remedy?

You must weigh the risks versus the benefits. See if there is any real data to support a remedy's claims, and investigate the possibility of dangerous side effects and interactions with other drugs.

Can alternative therapies really help?

In some cases, yes. But the effects of alternative therapies are highly variable. They may be a legitimate aid to some people, and have no impact whatsoever on others. A number of people find alternatives helpful due to their so-called placebo effect.

What is a placebo effect?

Mind-over-matter placebo effects take place due to the expectation or belief that a particular remedy will work. Placebos have no real effect on the body, but on average a third of people who participate in clinical trials feel better when they take them. In a study illustrative of the placebo effect, 13 people who were extremely allergic to poison ivy had one arm rubbed with a harmless leaf that they were told was poison ivy, while the other arm was touched with the real plant. The result? All 13 broke out in a rash where the harmless leaf had rubbed, while only two developed a rash from the actual poison ivy.

Is a placebo effect a bad thing?

Not unless it prevents you from following your regular treatment. Initially suspicious and dismissive of placebos, today many scientists have come to believe they are not such a bad thing after all. As long as a remedy is not harmful and makes someone feel better, it can function as a useful complement to more conventional approaches. A mistake, however, would be to substitute unproven remedies and the power of positive thinking for standard remedies that we know work.

Are alternative treatments ever harmful?

Yes. In recent years alternative remedies such as herbal remedies, acupuncture, and massage have exploded in popularity. Yet just because these are "natural" practices does not mean that they are inherently safe. For example, anyone can hang a shingle outside their door claiming to be a herbalist or nutritionist. But although dietary supplements such as herbs can, like regular medications, enhance your health, they can be very potent substances in and of themselves. In addition, herbs are subject to contamination and adulteration in their handling. Sensible safety precautions must always be carefully exercised when using any alternative approach.

Who seeks out alternative care?

A surprising four out of every 10 Americans are likely to turn to alternative remedies at some point in their lives. And a whopping 56% of those who seek out alternative care suffer from chronic pain such as that of arthritis, according to a 1993 study by the Kaiser-Permanente health care system.

I'm so exhausted that I can barely drag myself out of bed in the morning, and medications don't seem to do much for me. My doctor says that I have fibromyalgia. Can alternative remedies help?

Fibromyalgia is a syndrome of chronic pain and fatigue. Because it is so difficult to diagnose, this problem has traditionally been dismissed as an imaginary disease of "hysterical" females. Even though greater recognition is forthcoming (for example, the Arthritis Foundation recognizes that as many as 5 million people in this country suffer from fibromyalgia), it's no wonder that its victims often turn to alternative remedies.

Can alternative remedies really ease the pain and fatigue of fibromyalgia?

It's possible that techniques such as massage and acupuncture can relieve the aches and pains of this puzzling syndrome. To get the most out of either approach, give it a fair chance by scheduling a series of regular treatments with an experienced therapist. In addition, a good balance of rest and exercise and a healthy diet are essential. In particular, try to eat plenty of magnesium-rich beans, soy, seeds, nuts, whole grains, and green leafy vegetables.

What makes alternative care appealing to so many people?

There are many reasons. Most commonly, people seek out alternatives when conventional medical care just doesn't get the desired results. If you or a loved one suffer from chronic pain, you know how physically and emotionally draining it is. Since standard treatments rarely offer complete relief, frustrated individuals seek out possible alternatives.

What about managed care? Does frustration with this system play a part in the growing popularity of alternatives?

Most likely it does. The advent of managed care has meant that we receive less and less personal attention from a regular doctor, if indeed we are lucky enough to have one. It is probably at least partly out of frustration that many people turn to more caring alternative practitioners, who on average spend far more time with their patients.

What types of alternative care do Americans use?

In 1998, in a nationwide random survey conducted by InterActive Solutions of Grand Rapids, Michigan, people responded that they used these following therapies:

Herbal therapy	17%
Chiropractic	16%
Massage therapy	14%
Vitamin therapy	13%
Homeopathy	5%
Yoga	5%
Acupressure	5%
Biofeedback	2%
Hypnotherapy	1%
Naturopathy	1%

Should I consult with my doctor before trying an alternative therapy?

In most cases, yes. If you want to wear a copper bracelet or try a little meditation, go ahead. But before you try an alternative remedy such as glucosamine and chondroitin, be sure to consult with your doctor. Potential side effects and interactions with drugs you are already taking must be carefully taken into account.

What other precautions should I take before trying an alternative remedy?

- Make sure that you have a correct diagnosis of your problem.

- Tell your doctor about the natural remedy you are considering. Discuss its risks, benefits, and potential interactions with conventional drugs.

- Never stop taking your regular medication without first consulting your physician.

- Remember that *natural* is not synonymous with *safe*.

- Let the buyer beware. Maintain a healthy level of skepticism, for while evidence is mounting that alternative techniques can be helpful, there are still many quacks out there. If it sounds too good to be true, it probably is.

NUTRITIONAL SUPPLEMENTS

Are vitamins and minerals helpful?

Many scientists believe that a proper balance of vitamins and minerals can play a role in the treatment of arthritis. Do keep in mind, however, that supplements should be taken under your doctor's supervision.

Two supplements—glucosamine and chondroitin—have received a great deal of press in the last few years. Can they really help control the symptoms of arthritis?

In 1997, *The Arthritis Cure* was published to enormous acclaim. The authors—Jason Theodosakis, Barry Fox, and Brenda Adderly—recommend a nine-point program for osteoarthritis featuring a combination of two nutritional supplements: glucosamine (an artificially synthesized form of glucosamine, a substance that provides rigidity and strength to cartilage) and chondroitin sulfates (made from cow, shark, or whale cartilage).

What are the elements of *The Arthritis Cure*?

The authors recommend the following nine-point plan:

1. Have a thorough consultation with your doctor.

2. Take glucosamine and chondroitin sulfates to repair damaged joints.

3. "Improve your biomechanics" (use your joints the right way).

4. Get regular exercise.

5. Eat the right foods.

6. Maintain an ideal body weight.

7. Fight depression.

8. Take "traditional" medication as necessary.

9. Keep a positive outlook.

Will following this plan truly cure my arthritis?

No, because as you know by now there is no cure for arthritis. However, this program *does* make many arthritis sufferers feel much better. If standard remedies fail to control your pain and inflammation, ask your doctor if it would be appropriate for you to give it a try.

What about antioxidants? I've heard that they're good for arthritis.

Research suggests that people who have osteoarthritis are deficient in these valuable nutrients. Antioxidants such as vitamins A, C, E, and selenium can fight off free radicals and thus enhance your body's natural anti-inflammatory responses.

What are the recommended doses of antioxidants?

Although you should consult your own physician to determine the dosage that is right for you, the following are generally recommended dosages:

Vitamin A	5000 IU (International Units)
Vitamin C	500 to 4000 mg (milligrams)
Vitamin E	100 to 400 IU
Selenium	55 to 200 mcg (micrograms)

Are there any natural food sources of antioxidants?

Yes. Fresh fruits and vegetables are excellent sources of antioxidants. In June 1998, the University of California Berkeley *Wellness Letter* ranked blueberries as number one in antioxidant power. That is, blueberries finished first in the race to neutralize cell-damaging radicals. Strawberries, raspberries, and blackberries are also especially rich sources of phytochemicals such as anthocyandins and ellagic acid, antioxidants that help keep our cell chemistry stable. And in addition to their valuable antioxidant effects, anthocyandins may inhibit inflammation.

What about bioflavonoids? Are they helpful?

Yes. Bioflavonoids are naturally occurring chemicals found in plant foods. For instance, the anthocyandins in berries are bioflavonoids. These substances counter some of the effects of arthritis by supporting collagen and strengthening capillary walls, and they are also necessary for the metabolism of vitamin C. In addition to berries, green tea, whole grains, and seeds are good sources of bioflavonoids, which are also available in supplement form at health-food stores. In supplements, you will usually find them in combination with vitamin C, a multivitamin, or an antioxidant formula.

I've heard that fish oil can be beneficial. Is this true?

One to two teaspoons of fish oil on a daily basis can be helpful in managing inflammation, and research also suggests that omega-3 fatty acids can enhance the performance of the immune system. Do not exceed the recommended dosage on the supplement's label, however, since too much fish oil can cause problems with blood clotting. Fresh cold-water fish such as salmon, mackerel, sardines, and cod are naturally rich in omega-3 fatty acids.

Are dietary supplements safe?

Most are, but there's no way to know for sure. In the United States, dietary supplements sold in health-food stores do not have to be tested and approved by the FDA. In fact, they are not tested, approved, or inspected by any federal agency. The history of supplements is consequently rife with passing fads like melatonin. A few years ago, this hormone, ordinarily used to prevent insomnia, went flying off the shelves as a miracle cure for aging. (It wasn't.)

I'd like to try dietary supplements. What's the safest way of going about this?

Purchase dietary supplements from the most reputable sources you can find. For example, some well-known pharmaceutical companies are now marketing their own lines of supplements, and these may be your safest bet. The products of some smaller boutique companies may also be very good, but this you will have to find out from recommendations of others or by trial and error.

HERBAL THERAPY

What is herbal therapy?

Herbal therapy is the use of remedies prepared from roots, leaves, and other parts of plants for healing purposes. It is a holistic approach that emphasizes promoting health and preventing disease. Along with other alternative therapies, herbalism has become very popular as more and more people make the connection between body and mind.

According to herbal theory, specific ailments are the eventual outcome of both lifestyle choices and genetic predisposition. For example, even though we can't change the fact that OA is a fact of life for many of us as we grow older, there are steps we can take to prevent it from developing or worsening. In addition to taking herbs, these can include protecting your joints, doing regular stretching and strengthening exercises, controlling your weight, using heat and cold to relieve pain and stiffness, and remembering to pace yourself.

Are herbal remedies safe?

Many important questions about herbal safety have yet to be answered. In this country, herbal remedies are sold not as drugs but as dietary supplements. As a result, they do not have to be tested and approved by the FDA. Scientific trials of herbs have mostly taken place abroad, especially in Germany, where herbs are prescribed by doctors just like conventional medicines.

What is the difference between herbal therapy in the United States and in Germany?

In Germany, an agency called Commission E carefully evaluates the safety and effectiveness of herbs. Herbal remedies in Germany must be registered with the government and are standardized, so that you know exactly what you are getting. As of now, we unfortunately have no equivalent regulatory process in this country.

Is there any way to access the German research into herbs?

Yes. You can now access the helpful and reliable information from Commission E in the recently translated *Therapeutic Guide to Herbal Medicines from Commission E.*

What are some specific herbal remedies that I can try for my arthritis?

- **Curcumin,** the yellow pigment of turmeric, has very good anti-inflammatory and antioxidant properties. In one study of arthritis patients, curcumin proved to be just as effective as the prescription medication phenylbutazone in relieving swelling and stiffness.

- **Ginger** also has very good anti-inflammatory and antioxidant effects. When ginger is used in the treatment of both rheumatoid arthritis and osteoarthritis, studies have found that patients experience pain relief, decreased swelling and stiffness, and increased joint mobility.

- **Capsaicin,** a powerful substance derived from the cayenne pepper, is an active ingredient in many over-the-counter and prescription creams for arthritis. It works by depleting your body's supply of substance P, the chemical principally responsible for pain transmission.

- In one study, **devil's claw** was shown to relieve joint pain and reduce uric acid levels in gout patients.

- Other helpful herbs include **yucca, boswellia, ginseng, licorice, bromelain, bilberry,** and **feverfew.**

St. John's wort has received a great deal of media attention in recent years. Can this herb play any role in the treatment of arthritis?

St. John's wort may be helpful in the treatment of fibromyalgia. Because this herb can increase serotonin levels, it can help you get a good night's sleep and possibly even raise your pain tolerance.

Is St. John's wort a safe herb to use?

St. John's wort is generally a very safe and helpful herb when taken as directed. Occasional side effects include mild nausea, lack of appetite and fatigue, and one study indicated that large dosages may cause increased sensitivity to the sun.

In general, what safety precautions should I follow when using herbs?

Modern research confirms that herbs have a significant impact on the body, and plant remedies must be treated with the respect due to any medicinal substance. If you decide to give herbal remedies a try, here are a few basic safety guidelines to follow:

- Always consult with your doctor before taking any herbal remedy. While herbal remedies may complement medical care of arthritis, they are not meant to replace it.

- If you are taking COX-2 inhibitors or other medications, check with your doctor and pharmacist about possibly harmful interactions.

- Begin with the lowest recommended dosage of an herb, and increase gradually as needed.

- Do not exceed recommended dosages. Just because an herb (or drug) works well at one particular dose, this does not mean that it works better in larger amounts.

- If you are over 65, reduce the recommended dosages by 30%.

- If you are pregnant or nursing, do not use herbal remedies.

- If you suffer from other chronic health conditions such as high blood pressure or compromised liver or kidney function, consult with your doctor before using any herbal remedy.

- Stop taking an herb if you experience any adverse reactions, such as nausea, vomiting, diarrhea, or allergic reactions. If your reaction is severe, go to the emergency room of the nearest hospital.

- Always purchase herbs and herbal remedies from the most reputable sources you can find.

RELAX YOUR MIND

What emotional difficulties are associated with arthritis?

The pain, stress, and lifestyle changes brought about by living with a chronic disease can take a toll on arthritis sufferers. Some people lose self-confidence and self-esteem when no longer able to perform usual tasks, and others become depressed.

What are some good natural techniques I can use to relieve stress and control chronic pain?

Helpful methods include progressive muscle relaxation, tai chi, yoga, and visualization. The ability to relax and get a handle on stress is essential to pain management. Mind-body techniques such as meditation can help you achieve a state of deep relaxation.

What is deep relaxation?

The deep relaxation achieved via techniques like meditation and yoga brings about a variety of soothing physical and emotional responses. These include:

- Decreases in heart rate, respiration rate, blood pressure, muscle tension, and metabolic rate
- Decrease in general anxiety level
- A break in the cumulative effects of stress
- Increased energy level, productivity, concentration, and memory

Is meditation helpful for people with arthritis?

It can be very helpful. Meditation will not cure arthritis, but it can help control your symptoms by reducing your stress-hormone level, heart rate, and blood pressure. Many people begin to meditate for only five minutes at a time and find it so satisfying that they gradually extend their sessions.

What is the goal of meditation?

People who meditate achieve deep mental and physical relaxation while remaining awake and alert. Meditation helps you reach a state of inner and outer peace.

What is the cost of meditation?

Meditation is free. Moreover, it doesn't involve any drugs, and almost anyone can learn to do it.

Are there different kinds of meditation?

Yes. Three of the most popular forms are transcendental meditation, the relaxation response, and progressive relaxation.

What is transcendental meditation?

This type of meditation involves sitting quietly for about 20 minutes while your mind focuses on a sound, or mantra, while you breathe deeply. Concentration on a single word such as *Om* rids your mind of day-to-day concerns and helps you focus and relax. Another form of meditation is to direct your attention to a sensory memory, such as the heat of the sun on your body as you listen to ocean waves rolling onto the shore.

What is the relaxation response?

This is a similar technique created by Harvard cardiologist Dr. Herbert Benson, in which people choose a soothing word to focus on twice a day.

What is progressive relaxation?

Although there are many different types of progressive relaxation, begin with this simple exercise. Dim the lights and turn the answering machine down to make sure you're not disturbed. Close your eyes and relax. Search within yourself for any tension, and release it. Breathing in, visualize the muscles of the body, starting with your face. Breathing out, relax the face muscles. Gradually move downward, to the neck and shoulders, the spine, the arms, the torso, and the legs, consciously relaxing every muscle in your body.

What about breathing exercises? Can they help me relax?

Yes. Studies have found differences in the breathing of people who are relaxed and those who are anxious. When you are worrying about your arthritis and dwelling on its pain, you may notice that your breaths are more rapid and shallow. In contrast, deep breathing has a naturally calming effect on the sympathetic nervous system.

I'd like to try deep breathing. What do I do first?

At a quiet time in a peaceful place, try this simple exercise in mindful breathing. Slowly take a deep breath in, hold for a count of three, and exhale. Now simply sit quietly, resting one hand on your stomach, and feel your breath pass in and out of your body. Watch yourself breathe for the balance of the minute. If your mind starts to wander, gently draw it back. Just be aware of your breath: in and out.

What is biofeedback?

Biofeedback is another approach you can use to relax and help manage chronic pain. In this technique, small electrodes are placed on the forehead. Through them, electronic sensors measure your body's automatic functions, such as muscles that contract due to tension, breathing patterns, and pulse rate. As you practice different relaxation methods (for example, meditation), feedback from the sensors shows whether or not you are successfully relaxing muscles or slowing your pulse. The goal is to teach you how to consciously relax your own muscles, by watching and reducing the level of electrical responses on the gauge reading.

MASSAGE

Should I consider massage?

Massage, once considered solely an alternative therapy, is now practiced by mainstream physical therapists throughout the country. There are many different types of massage, which is thought to block pain signals from reaching the brain. Massage can be given by a professional massage therapist or you can give yourself a self-massage, stroking and kneading painful muscles that lie within your reach.

How does massage help soothe arthritic pain?

The kneading motions of massage increase circulation and warm painful areas. Massage soothes sore muscles and reduces tension in them.

What are the different types of massage?

Some are very vigorous and include pressing and tapping on the body. Others types, such as effleurage, are gentle. Special devices such as foot rollers, hand-held massagers, and shower attachments can provide relief too.

Are there any types of massage that I should avoid?

When you have arthritis, you should avoid deep muscle massage of painful joints. This can lead to further damage. Whenever you feel pain, the massage should cease immediately. In addition, do not massage swollen or painful joints.

MORE NATURAL REMEDIES

What about aromatherapy?

Aromatherapy is the art of using essential oils distilled from plants, flowers, fruits, and trees to enhance your well-being. Supportive aromatherapy treatments for arthritis include compresses, massages, and baths using essential oils. To relieve joint pain and inflammation, use essential oils such as rosemary and juniper to promote local circulation, remove toxins, and relieve swelling. Try a hot compress of rosemary, lavender, and arnica to relieve the pain of arthritis, or use these oils to massage aching joints. Alternatively, add a few drops to a warm bath.

Is acupuncture helpful in the treatment of arthritis?

Some arthritis sufferers find acupuncture helpful in alleviating pain, while others believe it enhances their immune responses. In this ancient form of Chinese medicine, specific points on the body are stimulated by very fine steel needles. The needles are then rotated by hand, or an electric current is applied to them. The goal is to balance the flow of *qi* or *chi* (pronounced "chee")—that is, energy or life force—along major energy pathways in the body called meridians. Although many people are initially intimidated by the idea of needles, the needles used are so thin that there is usually only minor discomfort.

Does acupuncture work?

It helps some people, although certainly not everyone. Scientists speculate that acupuncture works by stimulating the release of chemicals such as endorphins, your body's natural painkillers. It may also work in a similar fashion to TENS, which is a broadly accepted technique in arthritis treatment.

What is TENS?

TENS, or transcutaneous electrical nerve stimulation, is thought to work by distracting the brain from pain messages. Electrodes attached to the skin transmit a painless, low-voltage current. As a result, you feel a kind of tingling sensation.

Some fellow arthritis sufferers swear that magnets are helpful. Is this true?

Natural practitioners believe that magnets can be helpful in a wide variety of health disorders. They are said to relieve pain, inflammation, and stress, actions that would all be useful in the treatment of arthritis and related conditions. With the growing popularity of magnetic resonance imaging (MRI) in conventional medicine, it's possible that in time magnetic field therapy will gain greater credibility and more mainstream acceptance. In the meantime, if you want to try this therapy, consult your doctor first. Make certain that magnetic therapy takes place under the guidance of a qualified professional.

What is the story with the copper bracelets? Is there any basis at all to their reputation as an arthritis cure?

The fascination with copper dates back to Cleopatra and ancient Egypt. But while copper bracelets look pretty on your wrist (although they cause it to acquire a greenish hue), there is no evidence that copper cures arthritis or alleviates its pain and inflammation. If you'd like to wear a copper bracelet, by all means do so. However, also continue with your regular treatment.

What about bee stings and snake venom? Have people really tried these?

Yes. As you learned in the beginning of this chapter (or as you may have occasion to know from your own personal experience), people will try almost anything when they are desperate to relieve chronic pain. But you must look carefully into the pros and cons of a remedy before trying it. Is there any data to substantiate its claims? What about the risks of side effects or interactions with medications you are taking for your arthritis? Most importantly, talk to your doctor before trying any alternative remedy.

Glossary

Acupuncture—an ancient form of Chinese medicine in which specific points on the body are stimulated by very fine steel needles

Aerobic exercise—also known as endurance exercise, exercises such as walking, swimming, or bicycling which increases the flow of oxygen through your body, strengthening the heart and lungs, and improve overall fitness

Analgesics—medications such as acetominophen that are used to relieve pain but have no effect on inflammation

Ankylosing spondylitis—also known simply as spondylitis, or AS, this painful autoimmune disease causes stiffness and inflammation in the spine and joints in the extremities; in severe cases, vertebrae can eventually become fused

Antioxidants—nutrients such as betacarotene, vitamin C, vitamin E, and selenium that can neutralize some of the free radicals released during joint inflammation

Aquatic exercise—exercise performed in the water, which is an especially good choice for arthritic joints

Aromatherapy—the art of using essential oils distilled from plants, flowers, fruits, and trees to promote and enhance well-being

Arthralgia—achy joints

Arthroscopy—a minimally invasive surgical procedure in which a surgeon repairs joint damage through a small incision

Autoimmune disease—diseases such as rheumatoid arthritis and lupus, in which instead of defending against outside invaders such as viruses and bacteria for unknown reasons the immune system turns upon itself

Bioflavonoids—chemicals naturally occurring in plant foods that may counter the effects of arthritis by supporting collagen and strengthening capillary walls

Bone fusion—a surgical procedure in which two bones forming a joint are fused together to provide greater strength and stability

Bursitis—painful inflammation that affects small sacs called bursa, which ordinarily help muscles operate efficiently and easily

Carpal tunnel syndrome—a group of symptoms in which nerves pinched by swollen tissue causes pain in the wrists and numbness in the fingers

Cartilage—tough elastic tissue that normally covers the end of each bone in healthy joints, cushioning and supporting them

Celecoxib—the generic name for Celebrex

Chondroitin—in conjunction with glucosamine, a dietary supplement recommended in *The Arthritis Cure* which may be helpful in relieving the symptoms of arthritis

Collagen—a soft, supporting material that makes up almost three-quarters of bone

Corticosteroids—similar to hormones normally produced by our bodies, these medications can reduce the inflammation of arthritis; unfortunately, they have many potentially serious side effects

COX—a short-hand way of referring to cyclooxygenase, an enzyme that helps make prostaglandins

COX-2 inhibitor—a more selective sub-category of traditional NSAIDs (nonsteroidal anti-inflammatory drugs) which by inhibiting only the COX-2 enzyme relieves pain and inflammation without causing gastrointestinal problems

Cryotherapy—cold treatments to slow down nerve activity, relieve pain, and reduce swelling

Cyclooxygenase (COX)—an enzyme that helps make prostaglandins

DMARDs (disease-modifying anti-rheumatic drugs)—powerful medications which help to manage immune system activity and are prescribed to halt the progression of rheumatoid arthritis

Dyspepsia—stomach upset

Elimination diet—a diet eliminating specific foods one by one, for several weeks at a time, in order to determine if allergies are triggering symptoms

Endurance exercise—also known as aerobic exercise, exercises such as walking, swimming, or bicycling which increase the flow of oxygen through your body, strengthening the heart and lungs and improving overall fitness

Erythrocyte sedimentation rate (ESR or sed rate)—a measure of inflammation as indicated in a blood test; a high ESR indicates a high degree of inflammation, which may mean that you have rheumatoid arthritis

Fibromyalgia—a syndrome of constant, severe muscle pain and stiffness, disturbed sleep patterns, fatigue, and depression

Flares—periods when the pain, stiffness, and inflammation of rheumatoid arthritis are at their worst

Glucosamine—in conjunction with chondroitin, a dietary supplement recommended in *The Arthritis Cure*

which may be helpful in relieving the symptoms of arthritis

Gout—a form of arthritis caused by excess uric acid, leading to inflammation in joints such as the big toe

Herbal therapy—the use of remedies prepared from roots, leaves, and other parts of plants for healing purposes

Infectious arthritis—arthritis that is caused by an infectious agent such as a bacterium, virus, or fungus; Lyme disease is a form of infectious arthritis

Inflammation—swelling

Isokinetic exercises—isotonic exercises performed with the aid of machines

Isometric exercises—strengthening exercises in which you tighten your muscles and then relax them without moving your joints

Isotonic exercises—exercises in which you move your joints in order to strengthen your muscles

Joint—the place at which two bones meet

Joint aspiration—a procedure in which the doctor drains and examines some of the fluid from affected joints in order to make a diagnosis

Joint replacement—surgery in which severely damaged joints such as hips and knees are replaced with artificial joints

Ligament—strong rubberband-like connective tissue that holds the bones of a joint together

Lupus—also known as systemic lupus erythematosus or SLE, a potentially very serious autoimmune disease that affects the joints, organs, and skin

Lyme disease—a form of infectious arthritis caused by the bite of a deer tick

MRI (Magnetic Resonance Imaging)—used to diagnose arthritis and measure the extent of its damage

Nightshade vegetables—vegetables such as eggplant, potatoes, peppers, and squash to which some RA sufferers may be sensitive

Nodules—lumps that develop under the skin of rheumatoid arthritis sufferers

NSAIDs—nonsteroidal anti-inflammatory drugs commonly used to treat the pain and inflammation of arthritis

Occupational therapist—a medical professional who can teach you how to go about your day-to-day activities without placing undue stress and strain on your joints; they may also prescribe splints and other supportive devices

Orthotist—a specialist who designs and fits orthotic devices (such as braces and splints) to help reduce pain and inflammation by stabilizing weak or damaged joints

Osteoarthritis—the most common form of arthritis, in which wear-and-tear over the years leads to the breakdown of cartilage and consequent pain and stiffness

Osteoporosis—a bone-thinning disease that is a major cause of disability in older people

Osteotomy—a surgical procedure in which bone is cut and repositioned in order to correct a deformity

Paget's disease—a form of arthritis that produces excessive remodeling and overgrowth of bone, especially in the spine, pelvis, skull, and femur

Physiatrist—a medical doctor who specializes in physical rehabilitation and can design a comprehensive rehabilitation program for you

Physical therapist—a medical professional who can teach you how to perform exercises for greater strength and flexibility; they may also use treatments such as heat and ice massage, regular massage, hydrotherapy, electrical stimulation (TENS), and ultrasound to relieve your pain

Placebo effect—a curative effect that takes place not because a remedy has actual physical value but because the person taking the remedy has the expectation or thought or belief that it will work

Pleurisy—a symptom of lupus, pain in the chest when you breathe deeply that is unrelated to position or movement

Prostaglandins—hormonelike chemicals in the body that make nerve endings more sensitive and intensify the pain and inflammation of arthritis

Psoriatic arthritis—a condition related to ankylosing spondylitis, involving similar inflammations of the spinal joints

Purines—compounds found in foods such as organ meats and fish that are precursors of the excess uric acid that can lead to gout

Range of motion (ROM)—the extent to which you can move your arms, legs, or other parts of your body in any direction or at any angle

Range-of-motion exercises—exercises designed to enhance flexibility by helping you maintain and perhaps even increase the range of motion of your joints

Raynaud's phenomenon—a symptom of lupus and scleroderma in which fingers turn white and/or blue in the cold

Reiter's Syndrome—a condition related to ankylosing spondylitis, which involves similar inflammations of the spinal joints

Remission—periods in which symptoms recede and you feel much better

Resection—a surgical procedure in which all or part of a bone is removed to improve function and relieve pain

Rheumatoid arthritis—a severe autoimmune disease that causes stiffness, pain, and inflammation of the joints and often other organs as well

Rheumatoid factor (RF)—an abnormal antibody present in the blood of more than three-quarters of those who have RA

Sciatica—pain that occurs when back problems irritate one or both of the large sciatic nerves that extend down from the back, causing sharp or burning pain, weakness, numbness, and an uncomfortable pins-and-needles sensation in the legs

Scleroderma—a chronic, autoimmune disease of the connective tissue

Symptomatic ulcers—ulcers that cause pain

Synovectomy—a surgical procedure in which the diseased synovium (joint lining) is removed

Synovial fluid—the liquid produced by a joint's synovial membrane which allows bones to move without friction or pain; when synovial fluid is reduced by arthritis, cartilage is eroded and joints are damaged and possibly even destroyed

Synovium—the membrane lining the inside of joints

Tendinitis—inflammation of the tendons that attach your muscles to your bones

TENS (transcutaneous electrical nerve stimulation)—a therapy in which electrodes attached to the skin transmit a painless, low-voltage current believed to distract the brain from noticing pain

Thermotherapy—heat treatments such as hot water bottles and jacuzzis that relieve pain, promote circulation, and relax your muscles

Uric acid—a waste product that in excess amounts causes gout

Appendix A: Further Resources

Arthritis Foundation
P.O. Box 7669
Atlanta, GA 30357-0669
(800) 283-7800
www.arthritis.org

American Academy of Orthopedic Surgeons
6300 North River Road
Rosemont, IL 60018-4262
(800) 346-AAOS
www.aaos.org

Lupus Foundation of America
1300 Piccard Drive, Suite 200
Rockville, MD 20850
(800) 558-0121
www.lupus.org

National Osteoporosis Foundation
1150 17th Street, NW
Washington, DC 20036
(800) 464-6700
www.nof.org

Scleroderma Foundation
89 Newbury Street, Suite 201
Danvers, MA 01923

(800) 722-HOPE
www.scleroderma.org

Spondylitis Association of America
P.O. Box 5872
Sherman Oaks, CA 91413
(800) 777-8189
www.spondylitis.org

Appendix B: Further Information

BOOKS

Arthritis Foundation, *Arthritis 101*. Marietta, GA: Longstreet Press, Inc., 1997.

Brewer, Earl J., Jr., M.D. and Kathy Cochran Angel, *The Arthritis Sourcebook*. Los Angeles, CA: Lowell House, 1993.

Masline, Shelagh Ryan, The Johns Hopkins Health Series, *Back Pain: What You Need to Know*. Owings Mills, MD: Ottenheimer Publishers, 1998.

Schwarz, Shelley Peterman, The Arthritis Foundation, *250 Tips for Making Life with Arthritis Easier*. Marietta, GA: Longstreet Press, Inc., 1997.

Theodosakis, Jason, M.D., M.S., M.P.H., Brenda Adderly, M.H.A., and Barry Fox, Ph.D., *The Arthritis Cure*. New York: St. Martin's Press, 1997.

VIDEOS FROM THE ARTHRITIS FOUNDATION

- Pathways to Better Living with Arthritis

- PACE (People with Arthritis Can Exercise)

- Pool Exercise Program (PEP)

- Fibromyalgia Interval Training

- In Control (Arthritis Foundation Self-Help Course)

- Bone Up On Arthritis

Bibliography

Arthritis Foundation, *Arthritis 101*. Marietta, GA: Longstreet Press, Inc., 1997.

Sandra Blakeslee, "The Power of the Placebo," *The New York Times*, October 13, 1998.

Jane E. Brody, "Alternative Medicine Makes Inroads," *The New York Times*, April 28, 1998.

Shelagh Ryan Masline for The Johns Hopkins Health Series, *Back Pain: What You Need to Know*. Owings Mills, MD: Ottenheimer Publishers, 1998.

Shelagh Ryan Masline and Jason Elias, M.A., L.Ac., *Healing Herbal Remedies*. New York: Dell, 1995.

Shelley Peterman Schwarz for The Arthritis Foundation, *250 Tips for Making Life with Arthritis Easier*. Marietta, GA: Longstreet Press, Inc., 1997.

G.D. Searle & Co., Arthritis Fact Sheet. Skokie, IL: G.D. Searle & Co., undated.

G.D. Searle & Co., Celebrex Fact Sheet. Skokie, IL: G.D. Searle & Co., undated.

G.D. Searle & Co., Celebrex Press Release. Skokie, IL: G.D. Searle & Co., December 31, 1998.

Jason Theodosakis, M.D., M.S., M.P.H., Brenda Adderly, M.H.A., and Barry Fox, Ph.D., *The Arthritis Cure*. New York: St. Martin's Press, 1997.

Index

A

Ace-inhibitors, interaction
with Celebrex, 125
Acetaminophen, 75-76, 148
listing of brands, 75-76
Acupuncture, 265-266
benefits of, 266
Aerobic exercise, 158, 210,
214-215
aquatic aerobics, 220
beginning exercise, 214
benefits of, 215
forms of, 158, 216
walking, 214-215
Age, and arthritis, 9, 27, 38
Alcohol use
avoiding, 156-157, 181, 188
and gout, 171
Alendronate
for osteoporosis, 57
for Paget's disease, 58
Allopurinol, for gout, 85
Alternative treatments, 245-
250

acupuncture, 265-266
aromatherapy, 265
bee stings/snake venom,
267
copper bracelets, 267
effectiveness of, 245-246
and fibromyalgia, 247-248
herbal therapy, 255-259
magnet therapy, 266
massage, 263-264
most popular types of, 249
nutritional supplements, 251-
255
relaxation methods, 259-
263
safety of, 245, 247, 250
TENS (transcutaneous
electrical nerve
stimulation), 266
Alzheimer's disease, and COX-
2 inhibitors, 131
Analgesics, 30, 75-76
listing of, 75-76
over-the-counter drugs, 76
side effects, 76

Anemia, with arthritis, 34
Antacids, 194, 195
Antidepressants, 83-84, 149
  for fibromyalgia, 46, 83
  listing of, 83-84
Antioxidants, 185-187, 252-
  253
  benefits of, 185-186, 252
  food sources of, 186-187,
    253
  recommended dosage, 253
Aquatic exercise, 205, 209,
  217-220
  benefits of, 217-220
  forms of, 217, 220
  strengthening exercises, 218-
    219
  and water temperature, 219
Aromatherapy, 265
Arthritis
  and age, 9
  as chronic disease, 13
  diagnosis of, 15-18
  drug treatment, 142-150
  economic costs of, 20
  emotional impact of, 21
  forms of, 7-8
  gender differences, 8
  genetic factors, 11
  management of. *See* Pain
    management
  myths related to, 13, 15
  osteoarthritis (OA), 5, 26-
    32
  pain, causes of, 137-142
  prevalence of, 4-6
  prevention of, 12

  resources related to, 279-
    282
  rheumatoid arthritis (RA),
    5, 32-38
  social costs of, 20-21
  surgery for, 161-165
  warning signs, 9-10
Arthritis Cure, The
  (Theodosakis, Fox, and
    Adderly), 251-252
Arthritis Foundation, contact
  information, 233, 279
Arthritis-related disease
  bursitis, 42-43
  fibromyalgia syndrome, 44-
    46
  gout, 46-48
  low back pain, 38-42
  Lyme disease, 52-53
  osteoporosis, 54-57
  Paget's disease, 57-58
  scleroderma, 59-60
  spondylitis, 60-62
  systemic lupus
    erythematosus, 49-52
  tendinitis, 42-43
Arthroscopy, 18
  nature of, 164
Aspirin
  compared to COX-2
    inhibitors, 74, 118
  interaction with Celebrex,
    125
  listing of brands, 65-66
Autoimmune disease
  rheumatoid arthritis (RA)
    as, 5, 7-8

scleroderma, 59-60
spondylitis, 61
systemic lupus
erythematosus, 49, 50

B

Backache, 7
Back pain. *See* Low back pain
Bathroom, joint protection
guidelines, 238-239
Bedroom, joint protection
guidelines, 239-241
Bee stings, 267
Bilberry, 257
Biofeedback, 263
Bioflavonoids, 187, 253-254
benefits of, 187, 254
food sources of, 187, 254
Biopsy, 18
Blood tests, 17, 25, 34-35
erythrocyte sedimentation
rate (ESR), 35
for gout, 47-48
for lupus, 51
for red blood cell count,
34
for rheumatoid factor (RF),
34
Bone densitometry test, for
osteoporosis, 55
Bone fusion, nature of, 164
Boswellia, 257
Breastfeeding, and COX-2
inhibitors, 124

Breathing exercises, 262-263
breathing guidelines, 263
Bromelain, 257
Bursitis, 42-43
causes of, 43
management of, 43
signs of, 42-43

C

Calcitonin
for osteoporosis, 57, 88
for Paget's disease, 58
Calcium
daily requirement, 172
foods and absorption of,
173
food sources of, 172-173
for osteoporosis, 56, 56-57,
87, 88, 171-173
and Vitamin D, 172, 173
Cancer, and COX-2 inhibitors,
131-132
Capsaicin, 257
topical use, 90
Carpal tunnel syndrome, in
pregnancy, 35
Cartilage, functions of, 27-
28
Celebrex
and bursitis/tendinitis, 43
chemical formula for, 112
clinical trials, 100-107,
145
cost of, 126-127

Celebrex (*continued*)
counter-indications to use, 121-125
dosage, 31-32, 36, 127, 128, 232
drug interactions, 125-126
effectiveness of, 31, 110, 111, 118
FDA approval, 109-110, 145
and gastrointestinal side effects, 101-102, 119-120
and low back pain, 42, 130
overdose, 129
selectivity of, 116
and spondylitis, 62
and type of arthritis, 5, 25, 101, 110
See also COX-2 inhibitors
Children, and COX-2 inhibitors, 124-125
Chondroitin, 251-252
Cigarette smoking, and low back pain, 39, 41
Climate and arthritis, 14-15
Clinical trials, COX-2 inhibitors, 100-107, 145
Colchicine
for gout, 85
for scleroderma, 60
Cold treatments, 221-223
guidelines for, 160
ice applications, 222
safety guidelines, 222

Colon cancer, and COX-2 inhibitors, 131-132
Copper bracelets, 267
Corticosteroids, 31, 76-79, 196-197
bloating from, 196
counter-indications to use, 78-79
glucocorticoid injections, 79, 149
listing of, 78
mechanism of action, 77
and osteoporosis, 197
side effects, 77-78, 87, 196-197, 205
stopping/reducing dose, caution about, 197
Counterirritants, 90
COX-2 inhibitors
compared to aspirin, 74, 118
development of, 97-98
and form of arthritis, 5, 25, 36
future uses of, 129-133
for low back pain, 42
mechanism of action, 73, 98-99, 113-115, 115-116
Mobic, 6, 133, 148
compared to NSAIDs, 6, 70, 73-74, 99, 111, 113-119, 147-148
prevalence of use, 99
for spondylitis, 62
Vioxx, 6, 134-135
See also Celebrex

Creams. *See* Topical
  medications
Cryotherapy. *See* Cold
  treatments
Curcumin, 257
Cyclooxygenase (COX)
  enzymes
  COX 1, 72, 73, 113, 114
  COX 2, 72, 73, 113, 114,
    115
  NSAIDs effects on, 146-
    147
  role of, 72-73, 98-99,
    113

D

Daily activities, effects of
  arthritis, 20-21
Dental pain, 7, 130, 134
Depression
  and fibromyalgia, 44
  and pain, 139
Devil's claw, 257
Diagnosis, 15-18, 24-25, 30
  blood tests, 34-35
  diagnostic questions, 14-17
  and health care
    professionals, 18-20
  laboratory tests, 17-18
  time factors, 10-11, 28
Diet, 169-198
  alcohol use, 188
  antioxidants, 185-187

and arthritis, 15
bioflavonoids, 187
fasting, 191-192
folic acid, 195-196
food additives, 188
and food allergies, 189-
  192
and gout, 47, 48, 170-171
healthy diet, elements of,
  156, 179-185
and medications, 192-198
nightshade vegetables, 191
omega-3 fatty acids, 183-
  184
organic foods, 187-188
and osteoporosis, 171-173
vegetarian diet, 192
weight management, 174-
  179
Disease-modifying
  antirheumatic drugs. *See*
  DMARDs
DMARDs, 36, 79-82, 149
  counter-indications to use,
    82
  listing of, 81-82
  mechanism of action, 81
  side effects, 80
  for spondylitis, 61-62
Driving, comfort guidelines,
  242
Drug interactions, with
  Celebrex, 125-126
Drug treatment, 30-31, 36-37,
  142-150, 149
  analgesics, 75-76

Drug treatment (*continued*)
  antidepressants, 83-84,
    149
  corticosteroids, 76-79,
    149
  cost factors, 90-91
  COX-2 inhibitors, 6-7, 31
  DMARDs (disease-
    modifying antirheumatic
    drugs), 36, 79-82
  drugs with meals, 192-193
  fibromyalgia medications,
    82-84
  forms of, 30-31
  gout medications, 84-86
  muscle relaxants, 83-84,
    149
  nerve blocks, 149
  NSAIDs (non-steroidal anti-
    inflammatory drugs), 13-
    14, 24, 64-74
  nutritional effects, 194-
    196
  osteoporosis medications,
    87-88
  safety tips, 91-92
  topical medications, 89-
    90, 150
  tranquilizers, 149

E

Elimination diet, food
  allergies, 190-191

Emotions
  effects of arthritis, 21, 259-
    260
  and pain, 138-139
Endorphins, and pain relief,
  141-142
Erythrocyte sedimentation rate
  (ESR), inflammation
  indicator, 35
Exercise, 199-226
  aerobic exercise, 158, 210,
    214-215
  aquatic exercise, 205, 217-
    220
  beginning/frequency of, 210-
    211, 224
  benefits of, 30, 158, 199-
    200
  consultation with health
    care professionals, 205-
    206
  during flare-ups, 203
  and heat/cold treatments,
    221-223
  making time for, 202
  for osteoporosis, 56, 57,
    204-205
  and pain, 201-202
  range-of-motion (ROM)
    exercise, 158, 210, 211-
    212
  safety guidelines, 221
  strengthening exercise, 210,
    212-213
  sustaining motivation for,
    223-226

and weight management,
177-178, 215-216
yoga/tai chi, 158-159

F

Fasting, 191-192
Fatigue
and fibromyalgia, 44
management of, 140, 158,
160-161, 229
and pain, 140
and rheumatoid arthritis, 33
FDA approval, Celebrex, 109-
110, 145
Fertility, and COX-2
inhibitors, 123-124
Fever
and rheumatoid arthritis, 33
and systemic lupus
erythematosus, 49
Feverfew, 257
Fibromyalgia syndrome, 6, 44-46
and alternative treatments,
247-248
cause of, 44-45
diagnosis of, 45
differential diagnosis, 45
management of, 45-46
signs of, 8, 44
Fibromyalgia syndrome
medications, 82-84
listing of, 83
usefulness of, 82-83

Fingers, protection of, 236
Fish, in diet, 183-184, 254
Fluconazole, interaction with
Celebrex, 126
Folic acid, 195-196
food sources of, 196
Food additives, 188
Food allergies, 189-192
common allergens, 190
elimination diet, 190-191
relationship to arthritis, 189
Foods. *See* Diet
Free radicals, formation of, 185
Fruits, in diet, 182
Furosemide, interaction with
Celebrex, 125

G

Garden, joint protection
guidelines, 241-242
Gastrointestinal side effects
and antacids, 194, 195
and Celebrex, 101-102, 119-
120
death from, 122
and NSAIDs, 24, 25, 67,
68, 70, 73, 116-117, 143-
144, 194-195
prevention of, 68-70,
120-121, 144, 193
risk factors, 122
G.D. Searle & Co., 99, 131,
148

Gender differences
   arthritis, 8, 27, 33, 38
   osteoporosis, 55
   See also Women
Generic drugs, 91
Genetic factors
   arthritis, 11, 29
   lupus, 50-51
   osteoporosis, 54, 55
   spondylitis, 61
Ginger, 257
Ginseng, 257
Glucocorticoid injections, 79, 149
Glucosamine, 251-252
Gold. *See* DMARDs
Gout, 6, 46-48
   cause of, 47, 170
   diagnosis of, 47-48
   and diet, 170-171
   incidence of, 47
   management of, 48
   signs of, 8, 47
Gout medications, 84-85
   counter-indications to use, 86
   listing of, 85
   mechanism of action, 85
   side effects, 85-86
Guided imagery, 155

H

Headache, 7
Health care professionals, types of, 18-20, 206-207

Health insurance, coverage of drugs, 90-91
Heat treatments, 221-223
   benefits of, 223
   guidelines for, 159
   types of, 223
Herbal therapy, 255-259
   capsaicin, 257
   curcumin, 257
   devil's claw, 257
   in Germany, 256-257
   ginger, 257
   safety factors, 256, 259-260
   St. John's wort, 258
Hormone replacement therapy, for osteoporosis, 56, 57, 88
Hypnosis, 155

I

Imaging studies, and diagnosis, 17-18
Infections, and onset of arthritis, 12-13, 34
Inflammation
   and COX 1, 72, 73
   and prostaglandins, 72
   and rheumatoid arthritis, 10, 33
Internet
   arthritis-related Web sites, 279-280
   on-line support, 154
Isokinetic exercise, nature of, 213

Isometric exercise, nature of, 213

Isotonic exercise, nature of, 213

J

Joint protection, 157, 228-243
  in bathroom, 238-239
  in bedroom, 239-241
  body mechanics factors, 235-236
  and driving, 242
  for fingers, 236
  in garden, 241-242
  getting dressed, 241
  guidelines for, 228
  during household tasks, 234-235
  in kitchen, 236-238
  and movement, 228-229
  during travel, 243
  at work, 233-234
Joints
  damage from rheumatoid arthritis, 33
  joint aspiration, 18, 25, 30
  location of, 4
  specific joints and form of arthritis, 37-38
  stiffness, 230
  vulnerability to arthritis, 28, 29
Joint surgery, 37, 161-165

arthroscopy, 164
benefits of, 162
bone fusion, 164
indications for, 162
osteotomy, 164
physical therapy after, 165
pre-surgery guidelines, 162
recovery period, 164-165
resection, 164
risk factors, 162
synovectomy, 164
total joint replacement, 164
Juvenile rheumatoid arthritis (RA), drug treatment, 36

K

Kidney disease, and COX-2 inhibitors, 123
Kitchen, joint protection guidelines, 236-238

L

Laboratory tests
  diagnostic, 17-18
  See also Blood tests
Licorice, 257
Lithium, interaction with Celebrex, 126
Low back pain, 38-42
  arthritis-related, 40
  causes of, 38-40

Low back pain (*continued*)
  diagnosis of, 41
  management of, 41
  risk factors for, 40-41
  sciatica, 39-40
Lyme disease, 52-53
  and arthritis, 12
  cause of, 53
  management of, 53
  signs of, 52-53

M

Magnet therapy, 266
Massage, 263-264
  benefits of, 264
  types to avoid, 264
Meditation, 155, 260-261
  benefits of, 260-261
  transcendental meditation, 261-262
Menstrual pain, 7, 130, 135
Methotrexate, and nutritional status, 195
Mobic, 6, 133, 148
Muscle relaxants, for fibromyalgia, 46, 83-84, 149

N

Narcotics, 31, 143, 149
  cautions about, 76

Needleman, Philip, 97-99
Nerve blocks, 149
Nightshade vegetables, 191
Nodules, in rheumatoid arthritis diagnosis, 34
Nonsteroidal anti-inflammatory drugs. *See* NSAIDs
NSAIDs, 13-14, 24, 64-74
  counter-indications to use, 67-68
  compared to COX-2 inhibitors, 6, 24, 70, 71, 73-74, 99, 111, 113-119, 147-148
  dosage, 71-72
  effects on cyclooxygenase (COX) enzymes, 146-147
  lessening side effects, 68-70
  listing of drugs, 64-66
  longer-acting drugs, 69
  long-term effects, 70
  for lupus, 51
  mechanism of action, 72
  and nutritional status, 194-195
  over-the-counter drugs, 66
  pros/cons of, 116
  side effects, 24, 64, 66-67, 70, 73, 117, 143-144, 194-195
  taking with meals, 193
Nutritional supplements, 251-255
  antioxidants, 186-187, 252-253
  bioflavonoids, 187, 253-254

chondroitin, 251-252
daily multivitamin, 182
folic acid, 195-196
glucosamine, 251-252
omega-3 fatty acids, 185, 254
safety of, 254-255

O

Occupational therapist, role of, 19-20, 207, 209-210
Occupational therapy. *See* Physical/occupational therapy
Off-label uses, 112-113, 132-133
Omega-3 fatty acids, sources of, 184-185, 254
Ophthalmologist, role of, 19
Organic foods, 187-188
Orthopedic surgeon, role of, 18
Orthotic devices, benefits of, 157
Orthotist, role of, 20
Osteoarthritis (OA), 5, 26-32
   degenerative mechanism in, 5, 7, 10, 25, 27-29
   management of, 30-31
   prevalence of, 6, 26
   compared to rheumatoid arthritis, 37-38
   signs of, 9-10, 27
   See also Arthritis

Osteoporosis, 6, 54-57
   and corticosteroids, 197, 205
   diagnosis of, 55
   and diet, 171-173
   drug treatment, 57, 87-88
   features of, 8
   management of, 57
   prevention of, 55-56, 171-173
   risk factors, 54
   weight-bearing exercise for, 204-205
Osteotomy, nature of, 164
Overdose, with Celebrex, 129
Overweight
   and gout, 47
   and risk of arthritis, 12, 29, 174-175, 215-216
   See also Weight management

P

Paget's disease, 57-58
   management of, 58
   signs of, 58
Pain
   and antidepressant treatment, 84
   and COX 2, 72, 73
   and exercise, 201-202
   and fatigue, 140
   functions of, 141

Pain (*continued*)
  future uses of COX-2
    inhibitors, 130-133
  and joint stiffness, 230
  pain blocking mechanisms,
    141-142
  physiological causes of,
    137-138
  and placebo effect, 246
  and prostaglandins, 72
  psychological factors, 138-
    139
  and substance P, 90
Pain management
  drug treatment, 30-31, 36-37
  exercise, 30, 158-159, 199-
    226
  heat/cold treatments, 159-
    160
  joint protection, 228-243
  non-drug management, 32,
    37
  physical/occupational
    therapy, 14, 24
  and positive thinking, 150-
    151
  relaxation methods, 14, 154-
    156
  and sitting, 231-232
  social support, 154-155
  and standing, 231
  and stress management, 153
  weight control, 24
  See also Alternative
    treatments; Drug
    treatment
Pediatrician, role of, 19

Penicillamine, for
  scleroderma, 60
Physiatrist, role of, 19, 206-
  207
Physical/occupational therapy,
  14, 24
  post-surgical, 165
  compared to regular
    exercise, 208-209
  water exercise, 209
Physical therapist
  role of, 19, 207, 209-210
  treatments, 207-208
Placebo effect, 246
Platelets, and COX 1, 114
Podiatrist, role of, 19
Positive thinking, and pain
  management, 150-151
Posture, importance of, 231
Prayer, 155
Prednisone, for lupus, 51
Pregnancy
  and COX-2 inhibitors, 124
  and rheumatoid arthritis
    (RA), 35
  and systemic lupus
    erythematosus, 51
Prevention of arthritis, 12
Progressive relaxation, steps
  in, 262
Prostaglandins, actions of, 72
Psoriatic arthritis, 61
Psychiatrist, role of, 19
Psychological factors
  effects of arthritis, 21, 259-
    260
  pain, 138-139

Psychologist, role of, 20
Purines, high purine foods,
170

R

Range-of-motion (ROM),
meaning of, 25
Range-of-motion (ROM)
exercise, 211-212
benefits of, 158, 210, 211
types of, 211-212
Rash
and Lyme disease, 52
and systemic lupus
erythematosus, 49
Reiter's syndrome, 61
Relaxation methods, 14, 154-
156, 259-263
biofeedback, 263
breathing exercises, 262-
263
meditation, 260-261
progressive relaxation,
262
relaxation tapes, 156
Relaxation response,
262
Remission
and lupus, 50
rheumatoid arthritis (RA),
35
Repetitive movement, and
arthritis, 29
Resection, nature of, 164

Rheumatoid arthritis (RA), 5,
32-38
cause of, 7-8, 34
degenerative mechanism in,
5, 7-8, 10, 26, 33
diagnosis of, 34-35
joint damage, 33
juvenile RA, 36
management of, 36-37
compared to osteoarthritis,
37-38
in pregnancy, 35
prevalence of, 6, 33
remissions/flares, 35
signs of, 9-10, 33
surgery for, 37
and weight management,
178-179
Rheumatoid factor (RF), 34
Rheumatologist, role of, 18

S

St. John's wort, 258
Salicylates
listing of, 65-66
nonacetylated, 69
topical, 88-89
Salt, minimizing use, 181
Sciatica, 39-40
Scleroderma, 59-60
causes of, 59-60
diagnosis of, 60
management of, 60
signs of, 59

Sitting
    breaks during, 231-232
    and low back pain, 39
    at work, guidelines for, 233-
        234
Sjögren's syndrome, 19, 80
Sleep
    guidelines for nighttime,
        240
    problems and fibromyalgia,
        44, 45, 82-83
Snake venom, 267
Social support
    forms of, 21-22, 152-154,
        232-233
    support groups, 14, 22, 154,
        233
Social worker, role of, 20
Solanines, 191
Spondylitis, 60-62
    cause of, 61
    diagnosis of, 61
    differential diagnosis, 61
    genetic factors, 61
    management of, 61, 61-62
    signs of, 61
Standing, and pain, 231
Strengthening exercise, 210,
        212-213
    benefits of, 210, 212
    isokinetic exercise, 213
    isometric exercise, 213
    isotonic exercise, 213
    in water, 218-219
Stress, and fibromyalgia, 44-
        45

Stress management, relaxation
        methods, 154-156
Stretching. See Range-of-
        motion (ROM) exercise
Sugar, avoiding, 181
Support groups, 14
    benefits of, 14, 22, 154,
        233
Surgery. See Joint surgery
Swimming, benefits of, 219-
        220
Synovectomy, nature of, 164
Synovium, 33
Systemic lupus erythematosus,
        6, 8, 49-52
    cause of, 50-51
    and ethnicity, 49
    management of, 51-52
    signs of, 49-50

T

Tai chi, benefits of, 158-159
Tendinitis, 42-43
    causes of, 43
    management of, 43
    signs of, 42-43
TENS (transcutaneous
        electrical nerve
        stimulation), 208, 266
Thermotherapy. See Heat
        treatments
Topical medications, 31, 51,
        89-90, 150

advantages of, 89
hormone therapy, 56
indications for use, 89
listing of, 89-90
mechanisms of action, 88-89
Total joint replacement, nature of, 164
Tranquilizers, caution about, 149
Transcendental meditation, 261-262
Travel, comfort guidelines, 243
Treatment. *See* Pain management

U

Ulcers, preventive treatment, 69-70
Uric acid
drugs for control of, 84-85
and gout, 47, 170
high purine foods, 48, 170
Urinalysis, 17

V

Vegetables, in diet, 183
Vegetarian diet, 192
Vertebrae, fused, 62

Vioxx, 6, 113, 130, 133, 148
clinical trials, 134-135
effectiveness of, 134-135
Vitamin D, for osteoporosis, 56-57, 172, 173
Vitamins and arthritis. *See* Nutritional supplements

W

Walking, 214-215
water-walking, 220
Warfarin, interaction with Celebrex, 126
Water exercise. *See* Aquatic exercise
Water intake, daily requirements, 182
Weight machines, 213
Weight management, 24, 174-179
benefits of, 175
diets to avoid, 176-177
drinking water, 182
and exercise, 177-178, 215-216
health care professionals for, 175-176
and rheumatoid arthritis (RA), 178-179
Women
and fibromyalgia syndrome, 44
and rheumatoid arthritis, 27, 33, 38

Women (*continued*)
  and scleroderma, 59
  and systemic lupus
    erythematosus, 49, 51

Y

Yoga, benefits of, 158-159
Yucca, 257

HEALTH CARE BOOKS FOR THE INFORMED CONSUMER

SYNDROME X
Managing Insulin Resistance
By Deborah S. Romaine and
Jennifer B. Marks, M. D.
0-380-81444-7/$5.99 US/$7.99 Can

WHAT YOU SHOULD KNOW ABOUT TRIGLYCERIDES
The Missing Link in Heart Disease
by Dennis Sprecher, M.D.
0-380-80940-0/$5.99 US/$7.99 Can

CHOLESTEROL-LOWERING DRUGS
Everything You and Your Family Need To Know
by Richard W. Nesto and Lisa Christenson
0-380-80779-3/$5.99 US/$7.99 Can

CELEBREX ™
Cox-2 Inhibitors—The Amazing New Pain Fighters
By Shelagh Ryan Masline
Foreword by Jay Goldstein, M.D.
0-380-80897-8/$6.99 US/$9.99 Can

....

Available wherever books are sold or please call 1-800-331-3761
to order.
GEN 1101

**THE ACCLAIMED NATIONAL BESTSELLER!
OVER ONE YEAR ON *THE NEW YORK TIMES*
BESTSELLER LIST!**

WHEN BAD THINGS HAPPEN TO GOOD PEOPLE

HAROLD KUSHNER

Life-affirming views on how to cope with hard times and personal pain.

"Must reading for everyone who deals with tragedy."
Art Linkletter

"Provocative and comforting answers to the universal question: why me?"   *Redbook*

"A book that all humanity needs."
Norman Vincent Peale

"Harold Kushner deals with the theme of inexplicable illness with deep insight and provides invaluable reassurance."   **Norman Cousins**

0-380-60392-6/$6.99 US/$9.99 Can

Available wherever books are sold or please call 1-800-331-3761 to order.
KUS 1101

THE NATIONWIDE #1 BESTSELLER

the Relaxation Response

by Herbert Benson, M.D.
with Miriam Z. Klipper

THE CLASSIC MIND/BODY APPROACH
THAT HAS HELPED MILLIONS CONQUER
THE HARMFUL EFFECTS OF FATIGUE,
ANXIETY AND STRESS

81595-8/ $13.00 US/ $19.50 Can

00676-6/ $6.99 US/ $9.99 Can

Available wherever books are sold or please call 1-800-331-3761
to order.   RLX 0901